TURNING
POINT

TURNING POINT

The Myths and
Realities of Menopause

C. Sue Furman, Ph.D.

New York   Oxford
OXFORD UNIVERSITY PRESS
1995

Oxford University Press

Oxford   New York
Athens   Auckland   Bangkok   Bombay
Calcutta   Cape Town   Dar es Salaam   Delhi
Florence   Hong Kong   Istanbul   Karachi
Kuala Lumpur   Madras   Madrid   Melbourne
Mexico City   Nairobi   Paris   Singapore
Taipei   Tokyo   Toronto

and associated companies in
Berlin   Ibadan

Published by Oxford University Press, Inc.,
200 Madison Avenue, New York, New York 10016

Oxford is a registered trademark of Oxford University Press

Library of Congress Cataloging-in-Publication Data
Furman, C. Sue
Turning point : the myths and realities of menopause / C. Sue Furman.
p. cm.   Includes bibliographical references and index.
ISBN 0-19-508773-9
1. Menopause—Popular works.   2. Middle aged women—Health and hygiene.   I. Title.
RG186.F87   1995   618.1′75—dc20   94-16479

9 8 7 6 5 4 3 2 1

Printed in the United States of America
on acid-free paper

This book is dedicated to
my daughter, Laura,
and the young women
of her generation.

PREFACE

There are many turning points in a woman's life—puberty, marriage, birth of a child, birth of a grandchild, and menopause. Sandwiched in between are so many other events that perhaps on a smaller scale are in themselves turning points—first date, first kiss, high school and college graduation, first job, and the list continues. Most of these are approached with joyful anticipation and once passed are held as cherished memories. In the natural progression of a woman's life, it seems that menopause alone has stood as a turning point approached by many with anxiety and trepidation.

Menopause, one of the unique experiences of womanhood, has for centuries had a negative image based on myths and misconceptions held by physicians and the women they treated. At best menopause is more or less ignored and certainly not appreciated as a major milestone in a woman's life. These views are reminiscent of the ho-hum attitudes toward flowers that Georgia O'Keeffe sought to overcome with her paintings. O'Keeffe looked at small flowers and felt that most people took them for granted and failed to appreciate their beauty. She decided to take a flower and "paint it big and they will be surprised into taking a look at it." She considered the common poppy and painted *Oriental Poppies* in which she captured a level of beauty and detail missed by most. Georgia O'Keeffe brought about a new appreciation for flowers and in the process contributed to a turning point in American art. It is time for women to adapt the attitude of O'Keeffe. Let's take a closer look at menopause and paint it big so others will be surprised into seeing it as a natural life transition and appreciate it as a beautiful part of a woman's life.

The painting, already begun, needs to be carried to completion. In the last few years, the medical community has reached a turning point. Attitudes have changed and menopause is now viewed as the natural, physiological transition that it has always been. Many responsible and caring health-care professionals are leading the movement to improve health care for peri- and postmenopausal women. Attitudes about general health care for women are also changing. More government funds are being allocated to study diseases that affect women either disproportionately or differently than they affect men. Large numbers of women are finally being included in the research efforts designed to examine a number of these diseases and their potential treatments.

Women's attitudes about menopause are also at a turning point. Women are shedding their negative, anxiety-ridden views of menopause and recognizing it as a natural life passage. Baby boomers who made juggling a career and family the norm and put men in the delivery room are now approaching menopause. Once again they are a driving force for change as they openly ask questions about what happens to their bodies during and after the menopause transition. Their interest is in part responsible for the growing number of publications that have transformed menopause from a taboo topic to a household word. Spurred by the appearance of *Silent Passage* by journalist Gail Sheehy, menopause has become an acceptable subject for all forms of news and even entertainment media.

Now baby boomers and women of other generations want to know, in language they can understand, what causes strange feelings and sensations like hot flashes, night sweats, irregular menstrual cycles, fuzzy vision, migraine headaches, grumpiness, forgetfulness, vaginal dryness, uncomfortable intercourse, urinary tract infections, incontinence, the feeling that insects are crawling over one's skin, the appearance of a moustache, "extra" body hair, and thinning scalp hair. Women also have questions about osteoporosis, cardiovascular disease, and hormone replacement therapy and the lifestyle habits that can impact these concerns as well as general health.

I approached menopause with many of the same questions but found some answers available only in the scientific literature. Some questions remain only partially answered, because much research remains to be done. As I searched for the best currently available answers to my questions, it occurred to me that many women lack the time, access to journals, or the scientific background to sort through the vast number of scientific papers relating to menopause. This book is my attempt to share the information available in the scientific literature. Some facts are important, some are intriguing, and all are meant to ease the mind about the menopause transition. I have tried in layperson's terms to present a broad picture of how hormones and their interactions literally shape the phases of a woman's life—concentrating, of course, on the hormone changes related to menopause. I have also presented pros and cons of hormone replacement therapy, which is neither a panacea nor a poison. The last few chapters stress the important role that lifestyle habits like nutrition, exercise, and smoking play as women make the transition to the other side of menopause. The ultimate goal of this book is to provide useful information about the wide range of peculiar symptoms, sensations, and feelings that are very normal during the menopause passage so that each woman is prepared to thoughtfully discuss issues of concern with her own physician.

Hohenwald, Tenn.   C.S.F.
July 1994

ACKNOWLEDGMENTS

The completion of this book was greatly facilitated by the support and assistance of others. The time and knowledge that Dr. Lisa McAdams and Dr. John Williams shared with me as I worked on this project are deeply appreciated. The comments made by Dr. Joye Hood, Beverly Dyas, Nancy Stanley and Nancy's friends Pat, Marianne, Char, Anne, Janice, Angie, Candy, and Marilyn were very helpful and are gratefully acknowledged. The guidance and recommendations of my editor, Kirk Jensen, were especially valuable as were the endless enthusiasm and insightful suggestions of my daughter, Laura. Finally, I am indebted to my husband, Terry, for his exceptional patience and unwavering encouragement and support as I wrote this book.

CONTENTS

4 More Changes, 53

5 Menopause Before Your Time, 73

6 The Silent Epidemic, 95

7 The Heart of the Matter, 111

TO THE READER

This book is intended to offer general information about some of the hormone-related changes that occur during a woman's lifetime, especially those that impact on the menopause transition and the years beyond. The accounts of women facing menopause-related symptoms that are presented in this book are based on actual case histories or personal stories, but names have been changed to protect privacy. Most characterizations reflect problems common to many women and may invite identification with the personal difficulties of a reader. Remember, however, that every woman is unique and should seek the advice of her own physician for answers to individual questions, diagnosis of symptoms, and recommendations or prescriptions for medications. A physician should also be consulted before making dietary changes or starting an exercise program.

TURNING
POINT

1

The
Chemistry
of Love

What Are Little Girls Made Of?

Remember Henry Higgins, the exasperated professor in *My Fair Lady*? Amused and mystified by Eliza Doolittle, he considered the many differences between the sexes and wondered, "Why can't a woman be more like a man?" For centuries men have entertained similar thoughts in their attempts to understand female behavior and physiology. Most have reasoned from Henry's point of view and unsuccessfully attempted to rationalize women in terms of male emotions and behavior. Why are women so soft and shapely? How can creatures so appealing at times be so confounding and perplexing to the male members of the species? What are little girls made of that enables them to grow into women who are wonderfully different from men? The puzzling contrasts between women and men are due to the unique blend of a woman's hormones. This rare combination underlies many of the physical and emotional traits that are distinctly female.

The word *hormone* means "I arouse" and aptly describes the function of the chemical messengers that are produced in one part of the body but stimulate or arouse specific tissues elsewhere. The countless physical and emotional differences between women and men primarily revolve around two hormones, *estrogen* and *testosterone*. Both sexes produce these hormones but in very different amounts. The female body, mind, and emotions are fashioned by a special mix of hormones dominated by estrogen, sometimes called the "female hormone." Males, on the other hand, produce copious amounts of testosterone, the "male hormone," that shapes and integrates their anatomy, physiology, and thought processes. Hormones along with a myriad of other body chemicals influence sexual development and learning patterns, promote attraction between the sexes, and keep the reproductive organs and cycles running smoothly.

Love Is in the Air

During puberty and the adult years, hormones plus an array of additional chemical messengers play a role in the attraction between females and males. The initial magnetism between sexual opposites may be prompted by *pheromones*, a special class of hormones that are produced in one person but travel through the air to influence the behavior or physiology of another individual. These air-borne messages cannot be sent "at will" nor can they be directed at a particular receiver, but some researchers believe they can attract a sweetheart.

Scientists first studied pheromones in animals and concentrated some of the most intensive research on *sex-attractant pheromones* released by female moths. Possibly the first observation was recorded over a century ago by the French naturalist Jean Henri Fabré. He left a newly emerged *female Peacock moth* in a cage in his den one morning and returned in the evening to find the room teeming with *male Peacock moths*. Fabré's recorded account of the event reflects his astonishment, "Coming from every direction and apprised I know not how . . . forty lovers eager to pay their respects to the marriageable bride born this morning." Since this early observation, scientists have learned that special receptors on the antennae of a male moth can recognize the sex attractant pheromone of a female of the same species, sometimes as far as 7 miles away. Once the male detects the pheromone, he follows the trail of the airborne sex attractant to the female sender.

Sex attractants have also been found in many types of higher animals. A female dog in estrus is probably a more familiar example of the powerful allure of a pheromone sex attractant. Male dogs of all sizes and descriptions respond when a female dog's pheromones indicate that she is willing to accept suitors.

Less is known about sex-attractant pheromones in humans, but receptors for human pheromones are thought to be in or around the nose. When stimulated by pheromones, these receptors send messages to the brain and it activates other body systems. Human pheromones do not seem to have the immediate effect seen in some lower animals. Instead, their actions are probably more subtle and influence physiological and/or psychological behavior over a period of time.

Some scientists believe that *copulins*, a substance present in secretions from a woman's vagina, may lure human males. Perhaps memories of the effects of copulins or another yet unnamed pheromone prompted a brief note that Napoleon sent to Josephine from the battlefront over two hundred years ago. It read, "Ne te lave pas. Je reviens." which roughly translated means, "Don't wash. I'm coming home." Obviously, Josephine had an "aura" that Napoleon found quite appealing. Only more research can clarify the function of copulins and speculations about its role in attracting men.

Females are not alone in the ability to send chemical messages. Scientists have isolated two compounds from male sweat believed to be pheromones. These may act as sex attractants, influence the timing of the menstrual cycle, or affect females in some other way. One substance, *androstenol*, is said to smell like sandalwood and the other, *androsterone*, reportedly has the aroma of urine or musk.

It is interesting that, in women, the ability to detect certain kinds of smells is hormone dependent and is much keener near midcycle when the levels of estrogen and progesterone are high. This heightened sense of smell also coincides with the time of ovulation when the probability of conception is greatest. Perhaps at this time a woman can more easily detect "the essence of a male," possibly in the form of a pheromone.

Finally, it is fascinating that sex attractants of other species are quite appealing to humans. For example, musk, civet, and other ingredients commonly used in perfumes are derived from the glands of animals that utilize these secretions to attract mates. These "fragrances" so attractive to the species of origin are also alluring to many humans.

A Certain Smile

Pheromones give a new slant to sexual attraction, but romance is not sparked every time a few molecules of pheromone waft by on the breeze. If Anthony Walsh, author of *The Science Of Love: Understanding Love and Its Effects on Mind and Body* is correct, "Nature has wired us for one special person." Walsh does not believe that a person can love more than one other at a time. Choosing "Mr. Right" may be based on accumulated data. According to John Money, director of the Psychohormonal Research Unit at Johns Hopkins University in Baltimore, each person may have a love map in mind that defines the unique ideal partner. Characteristics for the love map come from people and experiences from childhood days. By adolescence, all the things one liked, or didn't like, are categorized and recorded in the brain's circuitry. Characteristics like a certain smile, soft brown hair, green eyes, strong hands, a neat three-piece suit, or the way your father told a funny story may fashion part of the love map of "the ideal mate." Of course, each individual's image of a perfect companion is unique—so unique in fact that no potential partner will ever have all the wonderful characteristics of the flawless sweetheart of a love map. Still, a women or man can become dazzled by one special individual who possesses several of the love-map traits.

When that certain smile does come along, at least some of the reactions that can lead to love are chemical. In the presence of Mr. Right, chemical reactions are set in motion and the brain is perfused with *phenylethylamine* (PEA) and probably the neurotransmitters *dopamine* and *norepinephrine*. These chemical cousins of amphetamines induce the euphoria so characteristic of love. That most happy feeling can last for quite a while, but it doesn't last forever. Helen Fisher, author of *Anatomy of Love, The Natural History of Monogamy, Adultery, and Divorce*, believes that over a period of two or three years, the body becomes used to the effects of PEA, and the smitten come down off cloud nine often with a case of "the four-year itch." It seems that the fourth year of marriage is the peak time for divorce in the 62 countries she has studied. She and others believe that a four-year bond may have been nature's plan to assure primitive women the protection of a mate during the first few difficult years of raising a small child. A second child born about three years after the first may extend the relationship another four years until the infamous "seven-year itch" strikes.

Many relationships outlast the slump in PEA in part because of the production of another group of substances called *endorphins*. These chemicals seem to increase in amount with the continued presence of the same partner. Unlike PEA, endorphins are chemically similar to the *opiates*— heroine, morphine, and opium. Endorphins are sometimes referred to as the feel-good substances because they function as natural soothers, are important in the relief of pain, and promote a sense of well-being and security. Endorphin production can be enhanced by various conditions in addition to amiable companionship. Their levels also rise, for example, with intense and prolonged physical activity creating the blissful state that long-distance runners describe as a natural high.

Oxytocin is yet another substance that seems to foster and be fostered by romantic relationships. A hormone long associated with inducing labor and influencing other events surrounding birth, oxytocin is now thought to also encourage mothers to cuddle their babies. Scientists believe that it may stimulate the same type of snuggling behavior between adult men and women and produce feelings of contentment and attachment. One report indicates that oxytocin may even enhance orgasms. Oxytocin levels increase three to five times during climax in men and may go even higher when women reach orgasm.

Passion by Design – Hormone Domination

Relationships and sexual function are nudged by chemical substances like pheromones, PEA, and oxytocin, and are spurred by the daily, monthly, and yearly ebb and flow of the "sex hormones" *estrogen* and *testosterone*. A woman's physical processes involving sex, like vaginal secretions and swelling labia, are controlled by estrogen, but testosterone, although dubbed the "male sex hormone," controls desire in both sexes. Men have about ten or more times the testosterone of women, but that doesn't mean they have ten times the sex drive. A man uses much of his testosterone to promote a beard, body hair, muscle mass, and other masculine characteristics. The relatively tiny amount of testosterone that a woman produces is sufficient to meet her physical needs and to dominate the mental processes that motivate her sexual desires and conjure up fantasies of intimate moments with a male companion.

This point was emphasized by Dr. Barbara Sherwin, director of the menopause clinic at McGill University in Montreal. She studied the role of hormones in female sexual function in a group of women with low estrogen levels. When a small amount of testosterone was included with estrogen replacement therapy, the women were more easily aroused sexually, had more sexual fantasies, and said they felt stronger and more energetic than when receiving estrogen replacement therapy alone.

The roles of estrogen and testosterone in sexual functions are complicated somewhat because their levels constantly rise and fall, orchestrating an ever-changing pattern of physical and emotional demands. Men and women both have a daily testosterone cycle that peaks each morning. Men may wake up ready to act on their hormone-prompted emotions, but women tend to be easily distracted from sensuousness by the demands of preparing breakfast, getting children off to school, or leaving for work on time. Women may also be more self-conscious than men about their early-morning rumpled appearance. Researchers find that most couples actually have intercourse around 11:00 P.M. when the house is quiet, daily demands are minimal, and testosterone levels are low.

The daily testosterone cycle is superimposed on a more or less monthly hormone schedule. In men, it affects physical characteristics like beard growth, which is heavier as the monthly testosterone level rises and lighter as it declines. Evidence suggests that testosterone also influences male emotions. One study charted the moods of a group of men submerged on an atomic submarine for months. According to researchers, emotions cycled from euphoric to mildly depressed on a four- to six-week schedule. Yet, when confronted with the data, the men insisted that there was no pattern to their emotions; they considered monthly cycles a strictly female characteristic.

Female hormone cycles are a little more obvious than those of men because they are punctuated by the menstrual period. During the first half of the menstrual cycle, estrogen is on the rise, making a woman feel good physically and emotionally. About midcycle, progesterone becomes more abundant. Researchers associate the second half of the month with flagging emotions and a tired, achy body. As menstruation gets underway, the cycle starts anew, perking up the spirits and the body.

Testosterone levels also change during the course of the menstrual cycle, peaking at about the time ovulation occurs. According to some studies, the surge in testosterone tends to make women feel sexier and up to six times more likely to have an orgasm. Having these feelings during the most fertile period of a woman's cycle may reflect an evolutionary advantage that increases the likelihood that woman will conceive. Some women are also more receptive to masculine attention just before and after the menstrual period. Heightened interest in sex at this time of the cycle may be stimulated by the drop in progesterone and is probably also linked to a cyclic decline in the neurotransmitter, *serotonin*, that reportedly suppresses sexual desires.

Testosterone peaks are not the same each day or even each month during the year. Men and women alike experience an upsurge in testosterone in the fall. According to Dr. Winnifred Cutler, daily and monthly testosterone levels reach an annual high each October, the prime month for making love and for successful conception. In late spring and early summer, approximately nine months after the annual testosterone surge, there is an upswing in the number of births recorded. In April, at about the time birth rates are getting ready to peak, male testosterone levels drop by as much as 22 percent. Theoretically, desire is at its lowest point. Like other patterns in the body's chemical cycles, the fall testosterone surge probably has an evolutionary advantage. Neuroscientist Dr. Bruce McEwen suggests that historically babies conceived in the fall and born in spring or summer when food was most plentiful probably had a better chance of survival than infants born in the fall or winter when food was scarce.

The mechanism that controls the yearly hormone cycles in humans is not known, but studies of similar cycles in animals may provide some clues. Biologists have determined that the hormone and mating cycles of many animals are influenced by seasonal changes in day length. Mating takes place during fall or winter when days are shorter, and young are born in spring or early summer when days are longer. The pattern is similar to the timing of the fall testosterone surge and spring birth peak observed in humans, but little is known about a direct influence of day length on human reproductive cycles.

Some interesting insights have been gained concerning the effects of day/night cycles on humans by studying shift-workers who reverse their activities by working nights and sleeping days. Flip-flopping days and nights causes a reversal of daily peaks and valleys in the hormone cycles according to Dr. Estelle Ramey, professor emeritus of physiology and biophysics at Georgetown University School of Medicine. Researchers do not yet know exactly what physiological changes take place, but numerous shift changes seem to be difficult for the body to handle. People who continually alter their day/night cycles tend to be sick more often and frequently experience a drop in libido.

Testosterone – The Assertiveness Hormone

The ebb and flow of testosterone apparently influence more than sexual desire and the coarseness of a man's beard. A number of researchers like Dr. James M. Dabbs, Jr., professor of psychology at Georgia State University in

Atlanta, also link testosterone to aggressive behavior. In man's evolutionary past, forceful conduct may have been a social plus that elevated a man to "leader of the pack" in caveman circles. Now, however, aggressive behavior is considered socially unacceptable if it is not appropriately channeled. Studies of men with naturally high testosterone levels indicate that they tend to be "sensation seeking" in their activities. They like to drive fast cars, play contact sports like football, or engage in other endeavors that most might consider risky. Not all men are able to direct their penchant for aggressive behavior into productive projects. Some high-testosterone males unfortunately get their thrills from socially unacceptable undertakings. Dr. Dabbs points out that most homicides and assaults are committed by males between the ages of eighteen and twenty-one. This is the age group with the highest testosterone level, and men in this category are much more likely to become violent when provoked.

By comparison, women have only a fraction of the testosterone present in males, but it is sufficient to impact on female behavior. Although women are not usually as volatile as men, there are distinct personality differences between women with high testosterone levels and those with low levels. Dr. Patricia Schreiner-Engel, at Mount Sinai Hospital School of Medicine in New York City, found that women with low testosterone levels asked their physicians few questions and were generally very agreeable patients. Women with high testosterone levels, however, were more demanding and wished to be involved in their own treatment. The association of the female testosterone level with assertiveness apparently carried over into other areas of life for the 30 patients in one study. Most of the low-level testosterone women had low-level jobs and lived with men. Women with high testosterone levels were career-oriented, and few lived with a male partner. Scientists are just beginning to understand the range of effects that hormones have on behavior. Hormones probably influence women in many subtle ways that can have major impacts on relationships, goals, and other lifestyle choices. Researchers do know that hormone activity relies on the ability of the body's cells to communicate with one another.

Body Language

The 60 trillion cells of the human body use the *nervous system* and the *endocrine system* as major communication networks for coordinating activities. The nervous system is an interconnected network that sends a combination of electrical and chemical messages along designated pathways or *nerves* to a specific destination. These messages must be delivered quickly, but generally do not need to last very long.

In contrast, the organs of the endocrine system—the *hypothalamus*, the *pituitary gland*, the *thyroid gland*, the *parathyroid glands*, the *endocrine pancreas*, the *adrenal glands*, the *thymus*, and the *gonads: ovaries* in females, *testes* in males—are scattered throughout the body. The endocrine glands make and secrete hormone messengers that are released into the bloodstream, which delivers the hormones to their destinations. The transportation system is slower than that of the nervous system, but hormone messages generally do not require a speedy delivery. Often it is more important that the message last over a long period of time. This is possible because a single hormone molecule can set in motion a cascade of events that greatly multiplies and prolongs its effects.

Each hormone carries a particular message from an endocrine gland to a specific type of *target cell*. A hormone can recognize appropriate target cells that have special *receptors* which are complementary to the shape and size of the hormone molecule. Hormone and receptor fit together like a lock and key to form a *hormone-receptor complex*. Once formed, the hormone-receptor complex changes the activity of the target cell to respond to the needs of the body. Some hormones activate a physiological response in only one type of *target cell* or *target organ* while others stimulate responses in a wide range of tissues. Estrogen, for example, influences over 300 body functions.

Hormones come in a variety of shapes and sizes but basically fall into three chemical categories—*polypeptide hormones*, *fatty acid hormones*, and *steroid hormones*. Polypeptide and fatty acid hormones combine with receptor molecules on the *surface* of their respective target cells. Formation of a hormone-receptor complex triggers changes in the biochemical activities inside the cell.

Steroid hormones like estrogen, progesterone, and testosterone are lipids and can slip through the target cell membrane and enter the *cell nucleus* where their receptors are located. Each steroid hormone-receptor complex has a unique shape that allows it to bind to a specific part of a chromosome and turn a particular gene or group of genes on or off. For example, cells of the endometrium of the uterus have receptors in their nuclei for estrogen and progesterone which play a role in the thickening of the uterine lining during each menstrual cycle. The hormones "turn on" different sets of genes that direct the activities necessary for organizing the growth and maturation of the endometrial lining. If fertilization does not occur, estrogen and progesterone levels fall, the genes are "turned off," and the endometrial lining is sloughed as the menstrual flow.

The Preset Mindset

The influence of hormones starts long before birth. The gender of a developing fetus is defined by its genetic makeup that directs the formation of ovaries or testes. The developing brain must also be characterized as female or male. There is a *critical period* during development when the hormone environment establishes the female or male gender-related blueprint in the brain. Scientists have found that all brains start with a female configuration, but significant differences exist between mature female and male brains. In most species, the critical period for sexual differentiation corresponds with the time when the gonads of the male are most active. The testes of the human male fetus are most active between the 12th and 22nd weeks after conception and again during the first 6 weeks of postnatal life. During the critical period, certain parts of the brain, especially the hypothalamus, become particularly sensitized to either estrogen or testosterone. If estrogen dominates during the critical period, the developing brain is *feminized* or retains a female scheme. During the critical period, high testosterone levels provided by active testes result in *androgenization* of the brain, meaning that a male pattern is established. Normally, the forming brain is imprinted with behavioral characteristics appropriate to the genetic sex of the developing individual.

Although males and females retain receptors for both estrogen and testosterone, there is a difference in the way that hypothalamic cells respond to the hormones. For example, Drs. Richard Whalen and J. Massicci of the University of California found that the cells of the hypothalamus of the female rat take up more estrogen and hold it longer than those of the male. Other animal experiments have shown that disruption of the androgenization or feminization process during the critical period can forever change the gender-related behavior of the animal. Castration of a male rat during the critical period removes the testosterone source and causes feminization of adult behavioral responses. Conversely, if testosterone is injected into a female rat during the critical period, parts of the nervous and reproductive systems are masculinized and later sexual behavior is influenced. The same experimental manipulations performed outside the critical-period time frame have no effect on development or later behavior patterns.

Female and male brains show other distinct differences that have not yet been directly linked to the events of the critical period. For example, scientists have observed a difference in the ease with which girls and boys learn and master different types of skills. Girls generally learn to read earlier and with less difficulty than boys. On the other hand, a recent study at Johns Hopkins University in Baltimore found that among top math students, boys outshine girls 13 to 1. This does not imply that boys never learn to read well or that girls cannot excel in math. It simply means that, *on average*, it is easier for girls to learn to read and for boys to develop math skills. These hormonally influenced tendencies also impact on some physical traits. Throughout life, women *generally* hear better and are *more likely* to sing on tune than males. Women also *tend* to be more adept at interpreting emotions from facial expressions.

The dominating presence of testosterone or estrogen during critical periods of development simply sets the stage for gender-related adult behavior patterns. Internal hormone levels and external environmental factors continue their influence through childhood and beyond. Researchers agree, for example, that religious, social, and economic influences in a person's external environment can be crucial in modifying hormonal influences. People with very similar biological backgrounds can be swayed by their social environment to choose divergent lifestyles ranging from celibacy to prostitution. Hormones are powerful influences, but they do not cast one's fate in stone.

Long past childhood, variations in the amount of estrogen in a woman's body continue to have an impact on characteristics as diverse as the senses, learning ability, and memory. On the surface, these traits appear unrelated to reproduction, but during the first half of the menstrual period when estrogen levels are high, women literally have keener senses of hearing, sight, taste, touch, and smell than during the last half of the cycle when estrogen levels drop. Learning also appears to be affected by the rise and fall of estrogen. Dr. Bruce McEwen of Rockefeller University studied the effects of changing estrogen levels on the brains of laboratory animals and found that the number of synaptic connections between brain cells decreases when estrogen levels are low. The cell-to-cell connections are reestablished when estrogen levels rise. The rise and fall of estrogen levels during each menstrual cycle apparently affect women in much the same manner. Learning is easier during the first half of the cycle when estrogen levels are high and becomes more difficult as estrogen levels trail off near the time of menstrual flow. Low estrogen levels during the menstrual cycle and menopause have also been linked to faulty short-term memory. A woman may frequently misplace small items like her car keys or experience other fairly harmless but annoying behaviors when estrogen levels are low.

Female by Default

Hormones and the messages they carry tend to get the lion's share of attention, but it is essential to appreciate the importance of hormone receptors. The amount of hormone present is irrelevant if there are no receptors to communicate the hormone message to its target cell. This lesson is unmistakable in the genetic disorder known as *testicular feminization syndrome*, called *TF syndrome* for short. Individuals with this disorder appear to be normal females at birth and develop as little girls for the first several years of their lives. At puberty, these youngsters mature as seemingly normal young women, but menstrual cycles never begin. It is the lack of menstrual cycles that usually brings a TF individual to the doctor.

A blood test of a TF sufferer will show low levels of estrogen but testosterone levels that are normal for a young man. A check of the chromosome makeup of the patient will reveal that the "young woman" actually has the genetic composition of a male, 46 chromosomes including 1 X chromosome and 1 Y chromosome. (Females have a chromosome count of 46 that includes 2 X and no Y chromosomes.) Amazingly, a genetic male develops as an "apparent female" because the individual lacks testosterone receptors. The appropriate gene to direct the formation of testosterone receptors is lacking or nonfunctional. Through childhood and adulthood a TF individual has normal testes, but they remain in the abdomen and never descend to the scrotum. The testes produce plenty of testosterone, but since no testosterone receptors are present, the hormone cannot communicate with its target organs. Estrogen, on the other hand, is present in small amounts (all males produce some estrogen) and estrogen receptors are present on target organs throughout the body. The organs respond to the only hormone they "hear talking." Female genitalia appear, and at puberty breasts develop as do all of the other "female" secondary sexual characteristics that estrogen promotes. Outwardly, the individual is a female who has always thought of herself as a female. Most TF patients choose to continue their lives as "sterile females." They remain infertile but otherwise have perfectly normal lives as women. TF is a truly extraordinary example of the importance of hormone receptors.

The Hypothalamus

Maintaining an intricate balance of estrogen, testosterone, pheromones, PEA, endorphins, and the other hormones and neurochemicals that rise and fall in rhythmic cycles through a lifetime seems like an overwhelming task. Researchers do not know exactly how the body accomplishes this complex chore, but the brain, especially a walnut-sized region called the *hypothalamus*, plays a key role in modulating the levels of many of these substances. The hypothalamus makes up less than 1 percent of the total volume of the brain, yet it produces hormones important in controlling reproductive activities, body temperature, heart rate, blood pressure, blood composition, and water and food intake. The hypothalamus also produces the hormones critical in initiating the change from young girl to young woman.

Long before the first menstrual cycle, at about age eight, higher centers in the brain kindle the process of sexual development by sending nerve impulses to the hypothalamus that signal it to start producing and secreting *gonadotropin-releasing hormone* (*GnRH*). Sergio Ojeda of the Oregon Regional Primate Research Center in Beaverton speculates that the hypothalamus does not secrete GnRH before puberty, because the necessary nerve connections from other brain centers are not in place until that time. Recent animal experiments emphasize the importance of GnRH and the prominent role the brain plays in the reproductive cycle. Anthony Mason and colleagues at Genentech, Inc., in San Francisco, found that a mutation that removes part of the gene for GnRH results in hereditary *hypogonadism* in mice. Animals with the mutation have underdeveloped gonads, are sterile, and do not mate normally. Genetic engineering techniques allowed Mason to introduce the normal GnRH gene into the genetic material of mutant mice. The resulting genetically engineered hypogonadal mice were "cured," mated normally, and produced offspring.

GnRH is important to normal reproduction because it prompts the nearby pituitary gland to release *follicle-stimulating hormone* (FSH) and *luteinizing hormone* (LH) that prod the ovaries to increase the production of estrogen and progesterone. In the young girl, estrogen levels rise only slightly at first, because hormone production occurs primarily during sleeping hours. Later, at about age ten, daytime levels of FSH and LH also rise and prompt a significant increase of estrogen that is responsible for the development of *secondary sexual characteristics*, including the growth of breasts and the appearance of axillary (underarm) and pubic hair. The body is transformed from a child to a young woman as the pelvis widens and deposits of body fat appear on the breasts, hips, and thighs sculpting the mature female body. A spurt in height around age 12 is orchestrated by *growth hormone*, or *somatotropin*, from the posterior pituitary gland, but estrogen also plays a role. Less noticeable are the growth and maturation of the Fallopian tubes, vagina, and uterus, but these organs also mature. It is during puberty that fluctuating levels of estrogen sometimes affect behavior and provoke emotional outbursts, earning estrogen the nickname, "the raging hormone." Maturation proceeds and hormone levels approach adult levels, stimulating *menarche*, the first menstrual period.

2

Hormone
Cycles

Timing the Menstrual Cycle

Strange as it may seem, honeybees have provided interesting insights into some of the factors that may affect the timing of a woman's menstrual cycle. The queen bee in a colony releases a pheromone called *queen substance* that suppresses the ovaries of the worker bees so that only she can lay eggs. Scientists first suspected that women might also emit a pheromone in 1970, when they observed a tendency for women who lived together (e.g., in a college dormitory) to have simultaneous menstrual cycles. The resulting conjecture, that a pheromone was responsible for synchronizing the women's hormone cycles, was reasonable considering the large body of evidence supporting the existence of pheromones in bees and other animals.

Recently, Dr. Winnifred B. Cutler, author of *Love Cycles*, and her colleague Dr. George Preti expanded on this information with an interesting experiment involving young women. The researchers collected underarm sweat from female volunteers and periodically daubed aliquots of it under the noses of 10 other female volunteers who had normal menstrual cycles. Another set of women who served as a control group had alcohol daubed under their noses. After three months, the menstrual cycles of the women exposed to donor sweat began to synchronize, but there were no significant changes in the cycles of the women in the control group. This work strongly supports the probability of female-to-female pheromone communication that affects the function of ovaries in other women by altering the timing of the menstrual cycle. Presumably the pheromone works by influencing a change in the rate or amount of hormone(s) the women release, but the precise mechanism is highly speculative. Why one woman's pheromones are "dominant" and possess the power to alter the cycles of other women is another puzzle that remains to be solved.

Males also send pheromones that influence the behavior and hormone activity of females in some interesting ways. Researchers have known for some time that male pheromones from a male mouse, goat, or sheep can accelerate the beginning of estrus or ovulation in females of the same species. Drs. Cutler and Preti set out to investigate the possibility of male-to-female pheromone communication in humans. For this experiment, male volunteers wore underarm pads from which the investigators extracted "male essence." A group of female volunteers—chosen because they had menstrual cycles that varied from 26 to 33 days in length—had the extract daubed under their noses three times each week. After 12 to 14 weeks, the menstrual cycles of these women changed, lengthening or shortening, to an approximate length of 29.5 days. It is interesting to note that Dr. Cutler has found that women with 29.5 day cycles have the highest fertility rates. A similar group of women served as a control but were exposed to alcohol instead of male extract. These women experienced no significant change in the length of their menstrual cycles. It appears that menstrual cycles can be influenced by pheromones from other females and also by pheromones from males. Exactly how pheromones affect the female reproductive cycle is unknown, although it seems clear that pheromone messages are "processed" by the brain, which in turn relays messages to the endocrine system, setting it in motion. Whether or not the pheromone messages somehow affect the release of GnRH remains to be seen. Pheromones are currently the focus of considerable research, but they are not the only external influences that can affect menstrual cycle timing.

Missing Periods

The bulk of evidence indicates that menstrual cycles are brain-driven events, but other factors including the ratio of lean muscle to body fat may influence menstrual cycle timing. There is definitely a profound change in this ratio during puberty. An adolescent girl has a five-to-one ratio of lean muscle to fat tissue, but, by menarche, the lean-to-fat ratio has leaped to three-to-one, a hike of 125 percent in only two or three years. What causes this dramatic change? Dr. Sarah F. Leibowitz of Rockefeller University believes it is related to food preferences prompted by hormone control. In her research, Dr. Leibowitz has found that before puberty, children prefer eating carbohydrates and proteins. Foods containing fats are not as tempting to youngsters. The preference for carbohydrates is driven by *Neuropeptide Y*, a neurochemical produced in the hypothalamus. The rise in estrogen during puberty prompts the hypothalamus to increase production of another neurochemical called *galanin* that controls the body's appetite for fat. Galanin production can be stimulated by other mechanisms but estrogen is the key influence during puberty. Not only do girls begin to eat more fat-containing foods during puberty, they also begin to store more fat. The increased production of galanin coupled with already significant levels of Neuropeptide Y set the stage for a teen to crave foods high in calories, fats, and carbohydrates like chocolate cake, ice cream, and French fries.

By the time a young woman reaches the end of the puberty transition, 28 percent of the body tissue is fat, and hormone production, menstrual cycles, and ovulation are typical of the reproductive years. Some researchers believe that attaining a body fat composition of approximately 28 percent may be necessary to maintain the proper balance of hormones essential for ovulation and menstruation to occur. They reason that a minimum fat level may be a biological safety device to ensure a successful pregnancy and childbirth. For a woman of average size, 28 percent body fat is a store of approximately 99,000 calories—an amount sufficient to nourish a fetus through pregnancy (50,000 calories) and to supply milk for a baby for a month (1000 calories/day).

Scientists critical of this line of thinking cannot deny the fact that women who drop below 28 percent body fat often stop ovulating and quit having menstrual periods, a condition known as *amenorrhea*. Amenorrhea is often linked to extreme weight loss caused by illness or eating disorders like anorexia. However, illness is not always the underlying factor. Amenorrhea also occurs in women on the other end of the fitness scale. The increasing number of women who exercise regularly have produced a large and growing group of women who stop ovulating and menstruating. For example, women who participate in gymnastics, ballet, intensive running programs, or similar activities sometimes exercise so strenuously that they alter their lean-to-fat tissue ratio dramatically. The change in body composition or some accompanying factor triggers *hypothalamic amenorrhea*. This common form of amenorrhea occurs when physical or emotional stress modifies hypothalamic function and too little GnRH is produced or the timing of the GnRH release is altered. Either change can keep the hypothalamus from initiating a new menstrual cycle. In addition, amenorrhea may be an outward sign of low estrogen production that can cause undesirable bone loss. This form of osteoporosis is another problem frequently suffered by young athletes.

Emotional factors that create tension in the body may also affect the function of the hypothalamus and alter the start of the next menstrual period. Some women find the timing of their period changed by a few days while others experience amenorrhea and miss one or more menstrual periods. For example, most women have at some time noticed a change in cycle timing due to sickness. Even a cold or the flu can be sufficient to disrupt normal menstrual cycle timing. Moving, traveling, starting a new job, or entering college are other emotion-packed experiences that can upset the regular menstrual pattern. Stresses of this nature generally result in temporary changes that affect one or maybe two menstrual cycles.

Amenorrhea is expected during pregnancy or following menopause, but missing periods at other times can signal serious health problems. Amenorrhea can also be caused by other physiological changes including problems in the uterus, cervix, vagina, ovaries, pituitary gland, or the brain. Anytime a period is missed, the body is sending an important signal that something is wrong. A physician can usually remedy amenorrhea by suggesting changes in physical activities and/or prescribing hormone treatment.

Hormone Cycles

Once begun, menstrual cycles usually continue in an unbroken progression for about 35 years unless interrupted by pregnancy. Cycle length can vary but about 30 percent of all women have a menstrual cycle that is 28 days long. For convenience, this is accepted as a standard, although the majority of women have absolutely normal cycles that last between 21 and 35 days. The menstrual cycle is often perceived in terms of the 5 to 7 day *menstrual period*. However, the beginning of the menstrual flow really signals that one cycle has ended and a new one is beginning. It is the outward evidence of the ongoing internal hormone interactions.

Each *menstrual cycle* is initiated by the brain and involves the interplay of the same hormones that triggered menarche. The *follicular phase* or first half of the cycle is set in motion when neurotransmitters stimulate the hypothalamus. Cells of the hypothalamus must have a built-in clock, because they respond to the neurotransmitter stimulation by secreting *gonadotropin-releasing hormone* (GnRH) in hourly pulses (every 60 to 120 minutes). The GnRH activates the nearby pituitary gland to release *follicle-stimulating hormone* (FSH) and *luteinizing hormone* (LH). These hormones are collectively called gonadotropins (gonad = sex; tropin = stimulus) because their primary target organ is the gonad (ovary or testis). Low levels of gonadotropins are released from the pituitary gland on a continuous basis, but the pituitary responds to the rhythmic hourly pulses of GnRH by releasing hourly pulses of gonadotropins.

Once in the bloodstream, FSH and LH travel to the ovaries where 10 to 1000 egg-containing follicles have begun to grow and mature. Researchers do not know why or how some follicles are activated and others are not. The developing follicles respond to FSH and LH by secreting *progesterone* and *β-17 estradiol*, one of the body's estrogens. The 200 to 500 micrograms of estradiol produced each day equal a quantity smaller than a grain of salt. This may seem insignificant, but β-17 estradiol is actually the most plentiful steroid hormone during the follicular phase of the menstrual cycle. As a matter of fact, it is the most plentiful form of estrogen throughout the reproductive years and affects the function of many body tissues. Estradiol and progesterone each have a role in stimulating cells of the endometrium of the uterus to grow into a thick lining capable of supporting a fertilized egg.

The growing follicles soon form balloon-shaped protrusions that bulge from the smooth surfaces of the ovaries, giving the almond-shaped organs a lumpy appearance. Shortly before midcycle, one developing follicle, possibly the largest or maybe the one in just the right stage of development, takes the lead. Its growth surpasses that of all the others, which regress. The "chosen" follicle continues to grow and cause an immense swelling on the surface of the ovary. Finally, the follicle ruptures, releasing the mature egg from the ovary in the process of *ovulation*. The other follicles that had begun to develop now wither after ovulation and the ovaries once again become smooth-surfaced.

Ovulation is the turning point in the menstrual cycle, signaling the beginning of the *luteal phase*. The length of the follicular phase that sets the stage for ovulation (midcycle) can be quite variable, but the luteal phase or second half of the menstrual cycle begins with ovulation and quite consistently lasts 14 days (plus or minus 2 days) and ends with the beginning of the menstrual flow. The remnants of the ruptured follicle are transformed into a new structure called the *corpus luteum* (yellow body). This body continues to produce some estrogen, but increases its production of progesterone, which controls the final maturation of the blood vessels and glands in the lining of the uterus in preparation for implantation of a fertilized egg. The corpus luteum also produces *inhibin*, which, along with estrogen and progesterone, signals the pituitary to stop releasing FSH and LH.

After ovulation, the egg is free in the abdominal cavity and moves toward the *infundibulum*—the open funnel-shaped end of the *Fallopian tube* or *oviduct*. The infundibulum does not directly contact the ovary, but its many cilia-covered fingerlike projections called *fimbriae* do wrap partway around it. Currents created by the undulating cilia help sweep the egg from the ovary surface into the cilia-lined oviduct. The egg is urged along the narrow passageway that leads to the uterus by muscular contractions of the oviduct and beating cilia that are present on many of the oviduct cells. It is during this journey that the egg can be fertilized. If the egg is fertilized by a sperm during the 48 hours following ovulation, estrogen and progesterone levels remain high to support the new pregnancy. The fertilized egg or *zygote* continues through the oviduct and becomes implanted in the *endometrium*, the spongy, glandular inner lining of the uterus. The endometrium of the hollow uterus is surrounded and supported by the *myometrium*, a thick layer of smooth muscle that contracts during labor, and the *perimetrium*, an outer covering.

If fertilization does not occur within 48 hours of ovulation, a different process occurs to reset the system for a new menstrual cycle. The egg loses the ability to unite with a sperm and the corpus luteum survives only 7 to 10 days before it begins to disintegrate. The declining corpus luteum produces ever smaller amounts of estrogen and progesterone until too little is present to maintain the recently formed uterine lining. Some of the endometrium is resorbed, but much of the tissue detaches from the uterus, the blood vessels rupture, and the tissue is sloughed and expelled through the vagina as the menstrual flow. The first day of menstrual bleeding is considered the first day of a new menstrual cycle. The average amount of blood lost during a normal cycle amounts to about one-quarter to one-third cup. In one study, different age groups generally lost similar quantities of blood with 15 year olds tending to have the smallest loss and 50 year olds the largest.

During the menstrual cycle, special receptors in the brain monitor the changing amounts of estrogen and progesterone produced by the ovaries and respond to the changes by appropriately modifying the amounts of GnRH, FSH, and LH that are released. Researchers do not know precisely how the communication system works, but they do know it is very complex. According the William Crowley of the University of Tennessee Center of Health Sciences, these influences are primarily indirect. Early in the menstrual cycle estrogen and progesterone levels rise and *inhibit GnRH release* from the hypothalamus. This decreases stimulation of the pituitary so less FSH and LH are secreted. Then, just prior to midcycle, the high levels of estrogen and progesterone *stimulate GnRH release* from the hypothalamus and also promote an increase in the number of GnRH receptors on the pituitary, making it more sensitive to GnRH. These factors work together to prompt a dramatic surge in the amount of LH secreted by the pituitary gland. After ovulation, the ovarian hormones once again seem to *inhibit GnRH release*. Near the end of the menstrual cycle, decreasing levels of estrogen and progesterone signal the brain that pregnancy has not occurred, and the hypothalamus initiates a new menstrual cycle.

Aches and Pains During the Menstrual Cycle

Some women actually feel a twinge of pain termed *mittelschmerz* at the time of ovulation. Occasionally, mittelschmerz manifests as mild to severe pain that can be quite unexpected and alarming. The pain is sometimes so intense that it sends a distressed woman to her physician or the emergency room. There are no serious physiological ramifications of mittelschmerz, and the pain can usually be controlled with ibuprofen.

About half of menstruating women are affected by *dysmenorrhea* or painful menstruation, commonly referred to as *menstrual cramps*. The condition troubles some women occasionally and others on a monthly basis. Most have mild to moderate symptoms, but about 10 percent of menstruating women are severely incapacitated by dysmenorrhea for one to three days if untreated. In fact, dysmenorrhea is so widespread that it is cited as the most frequent cause of absenteeism from work and school among young women.

Dysmenorrhea is caused by *prostaglandin F2α*, a substance secreted by some of the cells in the uterus. It is one of many prostaglandins—a somewhat heterogeneous group of fatty-acid-like substances secreted by a variety of tissues. Prostaglandins affect a variety of functions including blood pressure, body temperature, kidney fluid balance, activity of the gastrointestinal tract, constriction of lung passageways, and contractions of the uterus. The production of prostaglandin F2α by the uterus is under the control of the sex steroids. Its release during the menstrual flow stimulates uterine contractions that are responsible for most menstrual cramps. Women who experience severe cramps have four to five times the prostaglandin level as women who have a relatively normal and painless menstrual period.

Since the cause of menstrual cramps is known, physicians can offer remedies that are usually quite successful in alleviating the discomfort. Oral contraceptives are sometimes used to modulate the concentration of prostaglandins in the menstrual flow and control menstrual cramps. Other products like ibuprofen (Motrin), naproxen sodium (Anaprox, Naprosyn), and indomethacin (Indocin) reduce the amount of endometrial prostaglandins released by inhibiting the activity of *cyclooxygenase*, an enzyme that is necessary for the synthesis of prostaglandin. These medications are excellent for treatment of dysmenorrhea but may take several hours to bring relief. That makes it important to start medication at the first sign of discomfort. Cramping that is not relieved by ibuprofen or one of the other prostaglandin synthetase inhibitors may be a sign of more serious problem like endometriosis. This is often the case if dysmenorrhea begins several years after menarche.

When Getting Pregnant Is Difficult

The menstrual cycle is nature's design to repeatedly ready a woman to become pregnant. However, about 10 percent of the couples in the United States are unable to have children because one partner is *sterile*. Another 10 percent of American couples of reproductive age are *infertile* or unable to establish a pregnancy during a 12-month period. Common infertility problems of men include a low sperm count, compromised sperm-oocyte fusion, chromosome abnormalities, or other physiological problems, but sometimes the reason for infertility cannot be determined. A World Health Organization task force has reported that women frequently face infertility because of tubal factors (36%), ovulatory disorders (33%), or endometriosis (6%), but often there was no demonstrable cause (40%) of infertility.

A recent report from the National Center for Health Statistics stated that in 1988, 8.4 percent of women aged 15 to 44 were found to be infertile. That's a total of 4.9 million infertile women! Almost half of these women, 2.2 million, suffered *primary infertility* – they had no children. The rest, 2.7 million, experienced *secondary infertility* – they had one or two children but were having difficulty conceiving again. The startling rate of infertility is emphasized in a 1994 article in *The Lancet* in which researchers suggest that the rate of infertility among women is rising. The underlying cause may be biological. However, it is possible that the growing number of women who are waiting until they are in their less-fertile 30s or 40s to try to have children may be at least in part responsible for the trend. It is encouraging that doctors are now able to successfully treat many infertile men and women with hormones, corrective surgery, or techniques like *in vitro* fertilization.

The increasing number of women choosing to put off having children in their early years often to complete an education or pursue a career has created a challenging new frontier of having a child "against the odds." A woman's biological clock cannot be put on hold and continues to relentlessly tick away as goals are pursued. It is becoming far too common for a woman to finally fit pregnancy into her plans only to find that "when the time is right" her body is not ready. Some are faced with undiagnosed infertility in their 30s or 40s, and a few women decide they want to have a baby after their natural reproductive years have ended. Women in these situations are increasingly turning to hormone therapy, egg donors, and sometimes to surrogate mothers.

Women and physicians are now pushing the limits of infertility and menopause by artificially changing hormone cycles to extend the reproductive years. Surely one of the most remarkable surrogates is Arlette Schweitzer, the first American to give birth to her own grandchildren. Arlette's daughter, Christa, was born without a uterus but had functional ovaries. Many years later, Arlette gave Christa and her husband the gift of their own children. Arlette took hormones to nudge her body to prepare for pregnancy even though she was in the early stages of the menopause transition. Christa's eggs were collected and fertilized *in vitro* using her husband's sperm, and the fertilized eggs were implanted in Arlette's uterus. Nine months later she gave birth to her own twin grandchildren – a boy and a girl. Arlette appeared on the *Donahue Show* (June 17, 1994) and was asked about her attachment to the children she had carried. She revealed a very special attitude when she smiled and replied, "I was just the incubator. I'm not the mother, just the grandmother."

Interfering with the Hormone Cycle

According to Dr. Cutler, fertility is highest in women who have sex at least once each week and who have a 29.5 day menstrual cycle. Most women, including many who do not fit these criteria, do not have to struggle with the challenges of infertility. The hormones that regulate sexual desire and the menstrual cycle overlap so the appetite for intercourse peaks at the same time that ovulation occurs. This greatly enhances the likelihood of fertilization. Dr. Cutler has found that a woman has a 25 percent chance of becoming pregnant on her most fertile day. Nature's system to perpetuate the human species is so successful that it results in 230 births every minute. Since 90 people die each minute, there is a net gain of 140 new people every minute, which adds up to 1,400,000 new people every week or the equivalent of enough people to populate 52 new Philadelphias every year.

The majority of women contributing to the population growth are in their teens, 20s, or 30s. Most women nearing menopause no longer wish to have a new baby, but they should not rule out the possibility of becoming pregnant. Hormone levels can fluctuate for months or even years before menopause, causing menstrual cycles to be irregular and occasionally anovulatory (no egg is released). However, even a stretch of several months without menstrual periods does not ensure that menopause has occurred. Infertility rates are higher during these years, but pregnancy is possible even in the presence of irregular periods, hot flashes, or other menopause symptoms. Each year 3.5 million American women are surprised by an unintended pregnancy. Some of these are women who stopped using appropriate contraceptive methods, because they thought they were too old or too close to menopause to become pregnant. Contraception needs can change through the years, but this need remains until a woman has had no menstrual periods for at least one year.

Contraception or trying to interfere with the hormone cycle in order to prevent pregnancy has been a concern for thousands of years, simply because many women do not wish to be as fruitful as nature might permit. The earliest attempts at birth control were probably various forms of *pessaries* – devices or substances inserted into the vagina in an effort to prevent conception. Egyptian papyri dating from 1850 B.C. record the use of several pessaries. Some included acacia gum which may well have had spermicidal qualities. However, the most unique suggestion was the use of crocodile dung as a pessary. It is difficult to imagine what prompted the first application of crocodile dung, let alone its continued use. It probably was somewhat successful as a contraceptive, because it surely decreased sperm motility and may have had a spermicidal effect due its alkaline nature. Certainly, it is tempting to speculate that crocodile dung may have had an additional "aromatic power" capable of discouraging potential suitors.

During the seventh century A.D., Greek colonists founded the city of Cyrene in what is now Libya. They reportedly soon realized the contraceptive powers of a local plant called silphium. The plant's fame and the colonist's greed spread and by the third or 4th century A.D. silphium, which grew only in a small area, had been harvested to extinction. Other related plants continued to be used but proved much less effective than silphium. In the centuries that followed, different plants were employed for their contraceptive powers. Possibly the most notable was Queen Anne's Lace or wild carrot, which was revered by Hippocrates and others for its ability to prevent and terminate pregnancy.

Dioscorides, a second-century A.D. herbalist who served as an army doctor, described the preparation of drugs from plants for many uses, including birth control, in his work entitled *De Materia Medica*. His reported use of willow, date palm, and pomegranate as contraceptives may have had some validity. Studies performed in the 1930s indicated that material from all three plants decreased fertility in laboratory animals. However, their effectiveness in humans is not known. Dioscorides also suggested several other methods of contraception, including wearing amulets, asparagus, or cat testicles. These accoutrements may have dampened romantic urges, but they were otherwise ineffective methods of birth control.

Through the years, contraceptive techniques varied with the culture and the times, but never lacked for variety. Ancient Chinese women practiced *kong-fou* or total passivity in the belief that conception was not possible without orgasm. Of course, this was not true. Japanese women used a quinine pessary called *kijonomoto* or lady's friend. The *Kama Sutra*, written by Vatsyayana Malanaga, a fourth-century Indian physician, presented various methods of contraception including *coitus obstructus*. This technique involved squeezing the base of the penis in an attempt to force the ejaculate into the bladder to be expelled later. Albert the Great, a Dominican Bishop, added to the array of birth control practices by advocating drinking a man's urine or spitting three times into a frog's mouth. Modern birth control practices are more soundly based in science and use knowledge of the hormone cycles to avoid pregnancy. Still, some of today's birth control practices have long and interesting histories, as well as variable success rates.

On Your Best Behavior

Contraception has come a long way since the days of the crocodile dung pessary. *Behavioral techniques* are the simplest methods used today but are also among the least effective. Ideally, *complete abstinence* from sexual intercourse results in zero pregnancies. Realistically, 80 percent of the women who use abstinence as the only means of birth control become pregnant each year. The concept is great but does not take into account the ease with which idealism is forgotten in a moment of passion.

The *rhythm method* or abstaining from intercourse during the woman's fertile period (roughly days 10 to 20) is a little more efficient as a means of birth control. It is estimated that 2 to 30 percent of the women who use the rhythm method have unintended pregnancies. The concept of abstinence during a fertile period is thought to date back to Soranus, a Greek who practiced in Rome during the second century A.D. Unfortunately, he incorrectly believed that a woman's time of peak fertility coincided with the menstrual flow. Women who relied on this advice from Soranus probably had very large families. It was not until the 1930s that the fertile period was correctly determined to be near midcycle following ovulation. The efficiency of the rhythm method can be greatly increased if a woman is willing to keep accurate records of daily body temperatures (usually recorded on waking and before getting out of bed). Ovulation coincides with a body temperature increase of about 0.4° F and gives a fairly reliable indication that the likelihood of conception is very high in the days immediately following. In general, the rhythm method is an uncertain means of birth control because some women have irregular cycles and find record-keeping cumbersome.

Coitus interruptus or withdrawal of the penis before ejaculation is another behavioral technique with a long history. It was probably the most common form of birth control used during and after the Renaissance in the sixteenth and seventeenth centuries. The success rate is *estimated* to be as high as 75 percent but coitus interruptus is not very reliable as a method of birth control. Its effectiveness is severely limited by premature ejaculation and by the fact that small amounts of sperm-containing semen are often released prior to ejaculation. This can be a significant factor since one drop of semen from a healthy male contains between 5 and 10 million active sperm.

Spermicides

Spermicides or chemical techniques intended to kill sperm are commonly available today and have appeared throughout the history of contraceptive methods. An ancient Egyptian document, the Ebers Papyrus (1550–1500 B.C.), suggested using a tampon made of lint, honey, and acacia leaves to prevent pregnancy. The use of acacia is recommended in even earlier papyri. The long-term attention of the Egyptians to acacia apparently had some validity. Acacia can produce lactic acid, which has spermicidal qualities although its efficiency is not clear. Today spermicides come in an assortment of foams, creams, and jellies that must be inserted vaginally before intercourse in order to kill sperm as it enters the vagina. Spermicides are moderately efficient with an estimated failure rate of 15 to 20 percent. However, some failures can be attributed to using too little spermicide or forgetting to use the product at all. Then there is the very real likelihood that some sperm survive the chemical barrier and swim on to meet the egg.

Another chemical method, the *douche* or chemical washing after intercourse, was devised in the 1800s by Charles Knowlton, an American physician. Homemade and commercial douches are still available, but the method has been an unreliable form of contraception from the outset.

There was a period of time when most people including physicians associated contraception with prostitutes and women of low moral character. Indeed, for a while, the *British Medical Journal* believed the topic too disgusting to "soil" its pages. Accordingly, "ladies" were not given information about birth control by their physicians and women were forced to rely on word of mouth to pass along helpful contraceptive techniques. In the late 1800s, British women, concerned about the reliability of commercial pessaries, shared the recipe for "Contraceptive Fudge" in this manner. The ingredients and instructions for one batch were quite simple.

Contraceptive Fudge

Cocoa butter	1/4 pound
Borax	5 dram
Salicylic acid	1 dram
Quinine bisulphate	1 1/2 dram

Melt cocoa over slow heat. Stir in the remaining ingredients. When cool, cut into pieces and store out of reach of children.

This "fudge" was obviously not meant to be eaten. Instead, a piece was inserted into the vagina to serve as a pessary. While it may have had some spermicidal qualities, its effectiveness is not known. Today chemical techniques are often used in combination with physical barriers to improve the effectiveness of both.

Barricades for Sperm

Physical barriers like *diaphragms* and *condoms* are intended to prevent sperm from reaching the egg. The modern diaphragm is a flexible membrane that covers the cervix to prevent sperm from entering the uterus. It is reported to have about an 80 percent success rate. The effectiveness of a diaphragm depends to a degree on how carefully it is inserted.

Many forms of cervical caps preceded the diaphragm. In the 1700s, Casanova used a lemon half as a cervical cap. Casanova also reported an early type of condom that he called *Redingotes d'Angleterre* (English riding coats). He described them as "little preventive bags . . . to save the fair sex from anxiety." Condoms, originally introduced during the sixteenth and seventeenth centuries, were fashioned from linen and used primarily as protection from sexually transmitted diseases. Inventive individuals in the eighteenth century used 8-inch lengths of the cecum (a pouch-like portion of the intestines) of a goat, lamb, or sheep. History has it that the open end of the pouch was finished with a scarlet ribbon. Much later, the process of vulcanization of rubber allowed mass production of condoms and cervical caps that made contraception available to many.

Today, condoms fail at preventing pregnancy about 15 percent of the time because they leak, are put on incorrectly, or come off prematurely. Used not only as a method of birth control, condoms are also important as a means of preventing the spread of AIDS, herpes, and other sexually transmitted diseases. A female condom is also now available for contraception and as a barrier to sexually transmitted disease.

Sponges have been recommended as a physical barrier for contraception by many including the Marquis de Sade in his book *La Philosophie dans le Boudoir*. Sponges were originally intended to block the opening of the cervix and prevent the entry of sperm. Modern versions serve as a physical barrier, absorb sperm-containing semen, and also contain a spermicide. The effectiveness of the sponge depends on how carefully it is used. They are reportedly difficult to insert properly, which may account for estimates of effectiveness that range from 70 to 95 percent.

Although the *intrauterine device* (IUD) is inserted into the uterus to prevent pregnancy, it is not in the true sense a real physical barrier to sperm. How and why it works is not fully understood, but it somehow quite efficiently prevents the fertilized egg from implanting in the uterine lining. The success rate is a respectable 95 percent. Negative publicity from problems with an early model, the Dalkon Shield IUD, has quelled the use of newer and safer versions like the Copper T 380 IUD.

It is interesting that the "prototype" of the IUD was probably described by the Ancient Greek Hippocrates around 400 B.C. It was a hollow lead tube, filled with fat and inserted into the uterus to prevent conception. It appears that this "model" was never widely used. Somehow, it does not seem surprising that this particular device did not catch on as a popular method of birth control.

Pills and Injections

Since the 1960s, *birth control pills* that contain combinations of estrogen and progesterone have become popular. They work by preventing the maturation and release of an egg from the ovary during the menstrual cycle. Present-day birth control pills contain much lower hormone levels than those originally marketed. These newer versions are safer and have fewer side effects. They are also very reliable; fewer than 1 percent of the women who use the pill on a regular basis become pregnant in a given year. Research continues on a male birth control pill, but it is still in the future as a means of contraception.

Recently, the FDA approved the use of *Depo-Provera*, a new long-term birth control option that is 99 percent effective. It is administered by injection into the upper arm or buttocks once every three months. Each injection contains a synthetic version of progesterone packed in time-release crystals. The gradual release of progesterone sends a constant signal to the pituitary gland and depresses the release of gonadotropins. Depo-Provera is new to the American market but has been used by 11 million women in over 90 other countries. It is the choice of many who wish reversible long-term protection.

There are side effects, however. Preliminary evidence indicates a possible risk of breast cancer associated with Depo-Provera, but the FDA has reviewed numerous studies and believes the risk is minimal, if any. The drug does cause irregular menstrual periods and after two years of treatment about 80 percent of women stop menstruating totally. Some women *temporarily* develop symptoms of pregnancy like breast tenderness and nausea. Other problems include an average weight gain of four pounds per year for the first two years and an average delay of 10 months to regain fertility after the drug is discontinued.

The controversial French product *RU 486* or the morning-after pill is not yet available in the United States but may be in the future. How it works depends on when it is taken. If taken soon after intercourse, it prevents fertilization. If fertilization has occurred, it functions more like an IUD and somehow prevents the fertilized egg from implanting in the uterine lining. Some brands of birth control pills currently available can function in much the same way if multiple pills are taken at intervals during the 72-hour period following intercourse. Dr. Felicia Stewart, an outstanding advocate of family planning, is strongly in favor of this emergency birth control method. Physicians like Dr. Stewart and clinics like the student health center at the University of Texas at Austin have been administering this type of after-the-fact birth control for a number of years. When used later in the first trimester, after the fertilized embryo has implanted in the uterine lining, it is no longer considered a means of birth control. Instead, it is an abortifacient that is used in other countries to induce abortion during the first trimester.

In 1982, almost 16.5 million American couples reported *surgical sterilization* as their primary means of birth control compared to 10 million couples who used the pill. Surgical sterilization should be selected only after a couple is certain their family is complete since the procedure is very difficult and often impossible to reverse. In women, surgical sterilization involves *tubal ligation* or closing the Fallopian tube to prevent egg and sperm from meeting. In men, sterilization is accomplished by a *vasectomy* or removal of a small portion of each vas deferens (the tube that exits the testis) to prevent sperm from leaving the testes. The semen is normal in every respect except for the absence of sperm. Both tubal ligation and vasectomy are virtually 100 percent efficient at preventing pregnancy.

The number and variety of contraceptive methods available indicate the concern of many about having a reliable means of limiting family size. No single type of birth control is a panacea. Instead, each woman should discuss birth control with her physician and select the method that best suits her needs until she passes menopause.

3

Making Sense of the Menopause Myths

Symptoms of the Change

Hailed as "the female sex hormone," one might expect that estrogen, the hormone that "aroused" the reproductive organs at puberty and supported them throughout the reproductive years, would be sorely missed by them during the postreproductive years. That is certainly the case, but not the whole story. Scientists have found that estrogen does more than spur the reproductive organs through the childbearing years; it influences at least 300 body functions. Estrogen receptors have been found in many unexpected parts of the body: in several regions of the brain, in the nuclei of cells that stimulate bone growth, and in cells that line the arteries and capillaries of the circulatory system to name a few. The list of estrogen-sensitive tissues is long, and scientists continue to add to it. With this new information, some of the peculiar symptoms and sensations of the menopause transition are finally beginning to make sense.

All the symptoms that can occur as a woman approaches menopause are somehow related to the declining levels of estrogen. Some symptoms— night sweats, irritability, mood swings, forgetfulness, and concentration difficulties—particularly influence a woman's behavior. These and related topics are considered in this chapter. Chapter 4 addresses other estrogen-associated menopause symptoms including irregular menstrual periods, hot flashes, dizziness, headache, migraine, insomnia, palpitations, crawly skin, and visual disturbances. It also explains how declining estrogen levels induce changes in the reproductive organs that can result in vaginal atrophy, painful intercourse, incontinence, and urinary tract infections. In addition, Chapter 4 considers how decreased estrogen supplies can contribute to other obvious changes like dry skin and wrinkles, hair loss, and hirsutism (excess body hair). Subsequent chapters discuss how dwindling estrogen production elevates risks for heart disease and osteoporosis.

How many of these symptoms should a "typical women" expect? It is difficult to say. A few women, about 5 to 10 percent, breeze through the menopause transition and never notice any of the temporary symptoms commonly associated with impending menopause. Another group find themselves at the far end of the spectrum. They experience such severe distress from menopause-related changes that their quality of life is seriously diminished. However, the majority of women have one or a small number of menopause-related symptoms for a period of one to a few years. Women in this group generally view the peculiarities of menopause as annoying inconveniences and discomforts that can be quite unpleasant and exasperating but tolerable. Today, regardless of the severity of symptoms, there is no reason for any woman to "suffer through menopause." Estrogen replacement therapy can eliminate or at least relieve virtually all the symptoms of menopause. Alternative therapies are also available for those women with a history of breast cancer or other medical conditions that contraindicate taking estrogen replacement therapy.

Defining the Change

Menopause is a single event, a woman's last menstrual period. For most it occurs around age 51 and serves as a punctuation mark in the continuum of a woman's development. Menopause lasts about 3 to 7 days and is generally uneventful. In fact, menopause is so similar to every preceding menstrual period that it can only be identified in retrospect. By definition, a woman must experience a whole year free of menstrual periods before she can be certain that she has passed menopause.

The much longer interval of emotional and physiological transition that surrounds menopause is termed the *climacteric* (from the Greek word "klimakter" meaning "rung of a ladder"). This period of change roughly encompasses the years between 35 and 60 when a women experiences a continuing sequence of biological alterations as her eggs are depleted and her estrogen levels decline. Physiological modifications like the gradual loss of bone mass and the decline of the cardiovascular system are virtually imperceptible. They are, however, ongoing processes that proceed throughout the climacteric and continue for life. Unobtrusive in their progress, these alterations in the skeletal and circulatory systems can be devastating, because they sometimes culminate in potentially life-threatening consequences like broken bones, heart attack, or stroke.

The more obvious symptoms of menopause like irregular periods, hot flashes, and irritability occur primarily during a special part of the climacteric, the *perimenopause*, which more or less spans the two years prior to and the two years following menopause. Perimenopause is probably the period most women are referring to when they talk about going through *"the change of life."*

The climacteric, particularly the perimenopause, can be an emotion-filled experience that is profoundly affected by personal attitudes, self-image, cultural background, family, and social support groups. Today's perception of menopause and its influence on a woman's femininity, behavior, personality, sexual desire, and emotional well-being has been strongly prejudiced by historically negative attitudes and misconceptions. Concepts from the past associate menopause with physical and sexual decline, irritability, depression, and more. Some of the old beliefs are valid and should be recognized and understood. Others are myths that at best are founded on a small grain of truth. It is time to sort the realities from the menopause myths. It is helpful to understand the climate in which the myths arose and in doing so dispel the negative aura that has for centuries tarnished the image of menopause.

Menopause – Fact and Fiction

Historically, menopause was a mystery that was presumably enhanced because the event was rare. For centuries, life expectancy was so short that few women lived long enough to reach menopause. When the Roman Empire was in its prime (about 275 B.C.), the typical woman only lived to be 26 years old. Yet menopause was recognized as a natural if rare phenomenon for centuries. However, those who experienced menopause were surely very old by ancient standards.

It is estimated that the average age of the climacteric has remained unchanged since the 6th century A.D., making the average age of menopause almost twice the average life expectancy at that time. Life expectancy slowly crept up to 49 years of age by 1900. Women who passed menopause were not so rare but were still few in number and among the elders of the community. No wonder menopause has long been envisioned as the threshold of old age. For most of history, women who reached menopause had indeed outlived the majority of their peers. Furthermore, good nutrition and preventive health care were not well understood, so many "old people" had medical problems. The combination of factors made menopause, old age, and infirmity virtually synonymous.

In addition, myths, old wives' tales, and even early medical knowledge about menopause probably acquired a negative slant from misunderstandings about menstruation. Margaret Mead suggested that the sinister atmosphere long connected with the menstrual flow may have grown out of man's fear of blood. Hippocrates certainly characterized menstruation as a malevolent event when he proposed the widely accepted and long-held notion that the menstrual flow served to purge a woman's body of accumulated poisons. The explanation offered by Hippocrates was accepted as truth for centuries, but the concept of accumulating female poisons surely generated puzzling questions about menopause.

For a long time, the "debilities of menopause" were linked to the "female poisons" hypothesized by Hippocrates. What happened to "female poisons" after menopause? Did they accumulate within the postmenopausal woman and foster hot flashes, wrinkles, and other peculiar symptoms? Through the centuries, physicians concocted a variety of antidotes to cure the "miseries" that sometimes appeared about the time of menopause. The range of treatments peaked in the 1600s and 1700s when prescriptions included the benign (possibly enjoyable) remedy of drinking a glass of beer. Other cures were somewhat less palatable and ranged from eating raw eggs to ground animal ovaries. Surely the least pleasant remedy to relieve the distress of menopause was the practice of bleeding by leeches. No wonder women did not look forward to menopause. It loomed as the threshold of old age characterized by peculiar symptoms, and some cures were worse than the affliction. Menopause more closely resembled a millstone around a woman's neck than a milestone in her life.

Around the turn of the century and well into the 1900s, the negative image of menopause was enhanced by those in the medical community who painted a grim picture of the disposition as well as the emotional and mental stability of menopausal women. For example, Sigmund Freud cast menopausal women in a very dim light when he characterized them as "quarrelsome and obstinate, petty and stingy, sadistic, and anal-erotic." He apparently viewed the menopause transition on a par with the transformation of Dr. Jekyll to Mrs. Hyde. Freud was not the first, nor was he the last to perpetuate the myth that menopause transformed women into most unpleasant individuals.

Menopausal women were described in unflattering terms by a number of researchers including Emil Novak. In his 1923 edition of *Menstruation and Its Disorders*, he observed that, "The majority of women in the menopause have psychic symptoms. . . . They are peevish, irritable, morose, and depressed. . . . Many have full blown insanity with melancholia, paranoia, and maniacal conditions." Following this popular line of reasoning, physicians committed thousands of menopausal women to mental institutions with a "menopause-related mental disease" called *involutional melancholia*. Women diagnosed with involutional melancholia were characterized by excessive gloom, mistrust, and depression. Although the custom of institutionalizing menopausal women waned and is no longer practiced, involutional melancholia was not removed from the *Diagnostic and Statistical Manual of Mental Disorders* until 1980.

Negative characterizations of menopausal women continued and were fostered during the 1960s and 1970s by medical professionals like Robert Wilson, author of *Feminine Forever*. His beliefs were obvious extensions of medical dogma from years past. In a 1963 article about menopausal women he and his coauthor T. A. Wilson suggested that, "A large percentage of women . . . acquire a vapid cowlike feeling called a 'negative state'. It is a strange endogenous misery . . . the world appears as though through a grey veil, and they live as docile, harmless creatures missing most of life's values."

This description surely did little to generate a woman's enthusiasm for menopause, but Wilson's attitude toward the menopause transition was not unique. Instead, it reflected the thinking of the medical community of the 1960s. With the horrors of menopause well established, Wilson's real concern was "curing" women of their menopause ills using estrogen replacement therapy. He extolled it as a virtual fountain of youth in a pill that could restore a woman's former femininity. It is fortunate that more recent studies have dispelled many of the myths that arose long ago and persisted in the 1960s, 1970s, and even 1980s. Women no longer need fear being overcome by depression, infirmity, insanity, mania, or even "vapid cowlike feelings" as they approach menopause.

A New Image for Menopause

As late as the early 1900s, women nearing menopause were also approaching the end of their predicted life expectancy. The image of menopause has changed dramatically during this century. Menopause no longer looms as a reminder that a woman's remaining days are growing fewer, nor is it considered a disease. Thanks to improved nutrition and health care, female life expectancy has been extended to 79 years of age and is still rising. Not only are substantial numbers of women now experiencing menopause, today's woman can expect to live 30 or more years beyond menopause. Some experts are now predicting that a woman who is healthy at 52 will probably live to be 92. In fact, the Bureau of the Census and the National Institute on Aging predict that living to 100 will not be uncommon by the year 2050 when it is estimated that 15 million people or 30 percent of Americans will be aged 85 or older. To put it in perspective, many women who celebrate their 55th birthday in 1995 will be blowing out 100 candles in the year 2050! Americans are living longer, and views from the past that characterized menopause as the gateway to old age and debility are no longer realistic.

The future population increase in people over 85 years of age is presently reflected in the number of women passing menopause. Postmenopausal women now constitute the fastest growing segment of our society. Why the mass menopause? Baby boomers by the millions are entering their 40s. Today, 13 million American women are between the ages of 45 and 54; they are nearing or just past 51, the average age of menopause. Record numbers of women will continue to enter this age group that is anticipated to reach 19 million by the year 2000. In the face of dramatic increases in women's longevity and vitality, some still cling to the outdated notion that menopause and infirmity are synonymous.

Menopause is not an end. On the contrary, menopause is a new beginning—just as puberty, marriage, a career, motherhood, and all the other roles a women undertakes represent new beginnings. A woman can choose to be active, and practice good nutrition, exercise, and health care in order to nurture a youthful exuberance for life at 80, 90, and beyond. On the other hand, a woman can accept the myths from the past and expect to grow old and decrepit at 50. A woman tends to fulfill the self-image she pictures in her mind's eye. Accordingly, many aspects of the menopause transition are tempered by a woman's expectations, self-image, and attitudes that in turn are shaped by society and cultural background.

What Does 50 Look Like?

Dr. John Williams, a 30-year veteran of family practice medicine, says that the benefits of positive expectations and a positive attitude show through clearly among his many Amish patients. These women view menopause as a very natural part of life's continuum. According to Dr. Williams, his Amish patients have the least difficulty making the transition from the reproductive years to the postreproductive years. That doesn't mean that they never have hot flashes or other symptoms of menopause. Some do, but they stay active and confront symptoms in a positive manner and maintain a sense of humor that keeps the situation in perspective and their spirits high.

On the other hand, Dr. Williams observes that women who are concerned primarily with their physical appearance and who worry about "growing old" generally have the most troublesome perimenopause. These women picture menopause as a painful symbol of aging; they expect it to be bad. Women who believe menopause will steal their looks and usher in years of debility have the most difficult adjustment to make. They are brought face-to-face with the maturing process and a changing self-image. There is the stark realization that they cannot be 25 or 35 or even 45 forever. Unfortunately, women often get what they expect. Women who equate menopause with old age generally have the most aches, the most pains, and the most complaints.

Why are some women frightened of growing older? What does 40-something, or 50-something, or even 60-something look like anyway? It looks like Hillary Clinton, Candice Bergen, Dixie Carter, Rue McClanahan, Barbara Streisand, Carol Burnett, Lena Horne, Gloria Steinem, Elizabeth Taylor, Angela Lansbury, and many other stunning women. All are striking in their middle years. All are very active, and their many accomplishments reflect their self-confidence.

Even much older women remain remarkably lovely. Consider the birthday ladies that Willard Scott profiles on the *Today Show*. At 100+ years each has a beauty that radiates from her photo. Many send messages concerning their continuing activities that indicate their vitality and zest. There is a natural beauty that some women have after 50 that can continue past 100 birthdays. This kind of beauty reflects a woman who has matured and aged gracefully in contrast to one who has just grown old. As Dr. Williams observed, some aspects of menopause seem to be strongly influenced by a woman's self-image and her expectations.

What Do Women Expect?

In 1991, *McCall's* magazine surveyed postmenopausal readers concerning their experiences during the menopause passage. Most (66%) described a fairly smooth menopause transition, but about a quarter (25%) of the postmenopausal respondents said that menopause had been somewhat or very difficult. Premenopausal readers were also queried to determine their expectations about menopause. About half (49%) of the premenopausal women who participated said they looked forward to menopause as a positive experience that would free them from menstrual periods and concerns about contraception. The rest of the premenopausal women were less enthusiastic as they approached menopause. Some were resigned to menopause as a fact of life (27%), others preferred to ignore it (13%), and a few actually dreaded it (7%). The more negative attitudes are presumably colored by the historically negative image of menopause.

More than half of the women facing menopause thought the passage would provoke sexual problems (54%), cause mood swings (57%), and make it difficult to concentrate (64%). These problems can and do occur, usually during perimenopause. However, less than a third of the postmenopausal women who responded to the survey actually experienced sexual difficulties (22%), mood swings (31%), and concentration problems (24%). Obviously the concerns are real, but exactly what are sexual difficulties, mood swings, and concentration problems and how difficult is it to cope with them?

Still Sexy After All These Years

Wondering whether or not sex will change after menopause can create considerable anxiety for a woman. Yet from the 1800s until very recently, the medical community's care of postmenopausal women focused attention almost exclusively on the treatment of menopausal symptoms like hot flashes and "emotional problems." Little if any consideration was devoted to the sexual side of the postmenopausal female. There can indeed be physical hurdles like vaginal atrophy or recurrent vaginal infections that interfere with sexual pleasure (see Chapter 4), but these symptoms of menopause can be remedied with estrogen or other drugs. Some women may experience a slump in their desire for sex as their estrogen dwindles. This trouble can also be treated with estrogen replacement therapy. These are not insurmountable problems. They should be discussed with a physician and not allowed to hamper sexual activity and enjoyment.

Some of the myths about postmenopausal women and sex may be loosely based on facts. It is easy to imagine that in the years prior to modern lubricants and estrogen replacement therapy, women who experienced painful intercourse due to vaginal atrophy may have contributed to the myth that women lose their desire for sex at menopause. According to that myth, women supposedly respond to their lost sexual appetite by abruptly curtailing or eliminating sexual activity. The origins of this story are merely speculation, but Sigmund Freud, Robert Wilson, and other professionals promoted the idea fairly recently. Unfortunately, the myth persists today. Currently, a number of carefully performed studies are revealing the truth about the sexuality of postmenopausal women. Sex after menopause is often better than ever.

There are to be sure some postmenopausal women who are just not interested in sex. However, many of these women were not very interested in sex before menopause. A group of Danish investigators recently assessed the impact of menopause on trends in sexual desire and activity. They initially surveyed a group of 40-year-old women concerning their sexual activity. Then the researchers kept track of the sexual activities of the group of women until they reached age 51. The majority of the women (70%) experienced no change in sexual desire during the eleven-year period. However, *women who at 40 years of age anticipated decreased sexuality as a consequence of menopause found their expectations fulfilled* at age 51. This "negative anticipation" was the only single predictor of decreased sexual desire that the researchers observed. They concluded that women who are never very interested in sex will probably welcome menopause or any minor medical problem as an excuse to taper off or totally abstain from sexual activity.

On the other hand, women who have a satisfying sex life prior to meno-pause will probably maintain their sexual interest in the postmenopausal years. This has been verified by a number of other studies.

Dr. Edward M. Brecher, author of *Love, Sex, and Aging*, studied sexual-ity in a group of 4246 women and men over the age of 50 and found that many who are 50+ years maintain an active interest in sex. It is true that a comparison of the sexual activity of all men in the study to that of all women in the study revealed a clear decline of sexual activity among women. However, when *married women* were compared to *married men*, the levels of sexual activity were almost identical. Even among unmarried people over 70, Brecher found about two-thirds were still sexually active. In another study, Judy Bretschneider and Norma McCoy surveyed men and women aged 80 to 102 and reported that about half still felt sex was at least as interesting and important as it had been previously. According to Brecher, many people aged 50 and beyond find sex less intense than in earlier years, but it is often described as more tender and satisfying. He suggests that talking honestly and openly with a partner can lead to longer and more interesting foreplay or different positions for intercourse that can offset less frequent or slower arousal. Many researchers have also observed that it is not unusual for a woman to discover or rediscover climax after menopause.

Some women do find that sexual activity declines in the years after menopause, but not because there is a lack of interest. Sexual activities may diminish because a woman or her partner develop serious health problems. Other postmenopausal women find their sexual activity curtailed because they have no partner. In the late 1980s, life expectancy for women was 79 years of age while that for men was closer to 69 years. Many women are simply outliving their partners by a decade or more. Some women find new partners, but others do not. Starting over can be very difficult.

Most experts agree that a good way to find a partner is to stay active (or get active) and make new friends in social groups, church groups, or clubs where others share similar interests. "Dating" for the mature carries the same risk of rejection as it does for young people. In addition, mature adults can be dismayed by the disapproval of their children, friends, or even health-care professionals. Arno Karlen, long-time researcher and counselor in the field of human sexuality, urges the mature to, "Fight the stereotype that what was virile or sexy at 25 is lecherous or unseemly at 65. If ever there was an attempt to cheat the mature, it has been denying their need to physically love and be loved."

The Witches of Menopause

Freud, Novak, and others promoted an old notion that menopausal women become quite nasty. Fortunately, this is more myth than fact. A woman's personality is not transformed by menopause, but there are some physiological disturbances that can contribute to short tempers and mood swings. When hot flashes plague the nighttime hours, they are known as *night sweats*. A perimenopausal woman may be rudely awakened to find herself and her bedclothes drenched with perspiration. Night sweats can be distressing, and they can have far-reaching effects that upset daytime behavior.

Bouts of night sweats that rob a woman of proper rest night after night result in *chronic sleep deprivation*. The quality of sleep has been the focus of several studies. In one, the menopausal women who participated were divided into two groups. One group received estrogen therapy while the other received a placebo. The sleep patterns of all the women were monitored. The estrogen-treated patients took much less time to get to sleep, had fewer sleep interruptions because of night sweats or other reasons, and spent a greater proportion of time in dream-filled rapid-eye-movement (REM) sleep when compared to the placebo-treated group. Some investigators believe that a deficit of REM sleep can cause irritability and fatigue the following day. Others argue that lack of REM does not produce these symptoms. Researchers continue to debate the effects of disturbances during REM sleep and other periods of sleep. However, most agree that repeated interruptions of sleep from night sweats probably contribute to and may be primarily responsible for daytime irritability and fatigue. Menopausal women who are characterized politely as irritable grumps and less charitably as menopause witches may just need several nights of undisturbed slumber.

Sleep deprivation may also account for mood swings, feeling down in the dumps, or suffering weepy spells during the climacteric. Unexpected bouts of sadness can be just as distressing to a woman and those around her as uncharacteristic outbursts of temper. The underlying cause of mood swings is still being investigated, but the current best evidence indicates that in many cases these difficulties also stem from lack of proper rest caused by night sweats. Even women who do not wake up soaking wet (hot flashes and night sweats are not always accompanied by profuse perspiration) may have their sleep disturbed by body temperature variations and accompanying physiological changes. A woman who suffers from chronic sleep deprivation is much more likely to quickly change moods in situations she would take in stride if well rested. It is easy to speculate that irritability and mood swings related to night sweats fueled the myth that menopausal women are irritable, short-tempered, morose, and quarrelsome.

It is important to remember that irritability and mood swings are temporary changes in emotions that generally disappear after perimenopause. Many women quite understandably wish to feel better rested and want to control their emotional highs and lows by vanquishing night sweats before they finish the perimenopause years. Fortunately, night sweats, like hot flashes—their daytime counterpart, can be effectively managed with estrogen replacement therapy or somewhat less efficiently with clonidine and lofexidine (see Chapter 4). Repeated episodes of night sweats should be discussed with a physician to determine their origin since they can be symptomatic of some very serious diseases that have nothing to do with menopause.

Chasing the Blues Away

Sleep deprivation has nothing to do with an unanticipated sense of grief-like sadness that overcomes some women as they approach menopause. Instead, this despair arises when a woman has difficulty accepting the fact that she can no longer have a child. Even a woman who has completed her family and has no desire for more children may experience a sense of grief for her lost fertility. What provokes this unexpected melancholy? We only have clues as to the origin of this very real feeling. It is probably derived at least in part from social values of the past that equated fertility with femininity. For centuries, a woman's primary role was to have and nurture children. There is also a mystique connected with childbearing that makes most women feel very special. Today's woman is no longer defined by her fertility, but social and cultural influences may still color her emotions.

Grieving for lost fertility or suffering a short bout of the blues are not uncommon emotions during the climacteric. These are brief, temporary upsets. However, the old notion that menopause is associated with long-term depression is a myth presumably left over from Freud, Novak, and others who portrayed menopausal women as morose, gloomy souls. Numerous investigators have presented strong evidence to debunk the idea that depression and menopause are related. Dr. Karen Matthews, a professor of psychiatry at the University of Pittsburgh, followed more than 500 women for three years and found that those who had recently experienced menopause were no more depressed, anxious, or distressed than nonmenopausal women. Similarly, a recent study supported by the National Institute of Mental Health found that women between the ages of 45 and 64 had a lower incidence of depression than women in younger age groups. In a five-year survey of 2300 women, Drs. Sonja and John McKinlay, president and vice president of the New England Research Institute in Watertown, Massachusetts, found that 85 percent of the women reported no depression during menopause. The women who said they did have bouts of depression during the menopause transition numbered about the same as one would expect in the general population. The researchers found that menopause symptoms did not cause depression. Instead, women who were already depressed were more likely to report hot flashes and menstrual-cycle irregularities to their physicians.

These and other studies indicate that when depression does occur during the middle years it is probably triggered by other factors or life stresses that overlap the climacteric. For example, smoking, while unrelated to menopause, may contribute to depression that can occur during the menopause transition. A prospective study published in a 1993 issue of the *Archives of General Psychiatry* reports that women and men who are nicotine dependent are more than twice as likely to experience major depression than nonsmokers. The difficulty of coping with adolescent children during the premenopause years can also create stressful problems that underlie anxiety or depression. Other women reach menopause at a time when their children are older and leaving home. A woman who has centered her life around her family may suffer loneliness and anxiety from an "empty nest" when the children are no longer living at home. Then there are those women who find their lives disrupted by children who have been on their own and move back home—sometimes with children of their own. For some, an overcrowded nest can create as much stress as an empty nest. The most recent trend along these lines is characterized by children who drop grandchildren off to be raised by grandparents. This phenomenon has become so widespread that the American Association of Retired Persons (AARP) recently started a hotline for grandparents who find themselves in this situation.

Data from the Massachusetts Women's Health Study indicate that children are a primary source of worry during the climacteric, but they are not the only cause of anxiety. More and more women simultaneously face menopause and the challenge of caring for aging and ailing parents, a husband with health problems, or the death of a loved one – possibly a husband. For others, marital problems arise or culminate in divorce during the menopause years. Many problems that are unrelated to menopause but overlap the menopause transition can foster anxiety, tension, or even depression. However, these problems are coincidental with menopause, not caused by it.

The Absent-Minded Woman

Difficulty concentrating and short-term memory loss are two very real symptoms that are high on the list of concerns expressed by women approaching menopause. A short attention span or a faulty memory can be a major nuisance, but these are only temporary consequences of the climacteric. How do they affect a woman? Usually in exasperating small ways. Impaired concentration may make it difficult to balance a bank statement or check an income tax return. Absent-mindedness may cause a woman to misplace her reading glasses with some frequency or forget her grocery list when she goes shopping. How are these peculiar changes in behavior related to menopause? Temporary short attention span and absent-mindedness both appear to be promoted by decreased levels of estrogen.

The low estrogen levels that are characteristic of postmenopausal women apparently cause some synaptic pathways (nerve-to-nerve connections) in the brain to be disconnected. This type of breakdown in nerve-to-nerve communication in humans is probably similar to that observed in animals by Dr. Bruce McEwen of Rockefeller University. He found that animals with low estrogen levels also had decreased numbers of synaptic connections in their brains. Treating the animals with estrogen restored the synaptic connections. Similarly, estrogen replacement therapy "restores" concentration powers and short-term memory in postmenopausal women. No one knows why, but, given some time, these estrogen-induced lapses of mental focus and memory also reverse naturally with no treatment.

Of greater concern is new evidence indicating that low estrogen levels may play a role in Alzheimer's disease – the fourth most common cause of death in people over 75 years of age. Alzheimer's disease affects 4 million Americans and is almost twice as common in women as in men. It occurs almost exclusively in the years after menopause. It is interesting to speculate that postmenopausal women with Alzheimer's disease or other forms of senile dementia may have given credence to the menopause myth that depicted women as mentally unstable. Such conditions may have also contributed to the diagnosis of involutional melancholia that resulted in so many women being institutionalized after menopause.

The cause of Alzheimer's disease is unknown, but certain recently identified genes may increase the risk of Alzheimer's and lower the age when a person is affected. These genes are not the sole cause of the disorder, and therefore lacking the genes does not guarantee immunity from Alzheimer's. Early Alzheimer's, which may begin in a person's 40s, affects about 5 percent of all Alzheimer's patients and is linked to genes on chromosomes 14 and 21. Late-onset Alzheimer's, which affects the vast majority of sufferers, has recently been linked to a version of a gene on chromosome 19 that codes for *apolipoprotein E* or *apo E*, a protein that helps shuttle cholesterol in the blood. Only one form of the gene, *APOE-4*, is related to Alzheimer's. A person who lacks this gene is not exempt from the disease but is at lower risk than a person who carries one copy (4-fold risk) or two copies (8-fold risk) of the APOE-4 gene. The gene also impacts on the average age of onset of Alzheimer's. Those with two APOE-4 genes usually develop Alzheimer's by age 68 while patients with one or no copies of the gene do not usually succumb to the disease until age 75 or 84, respectively.

Diagnosis of Alzheimer's disease is problematic because the symptoms are similar to those of a number of other conditions. In fact, diagnosis can only be made with certainty from brain tissue taken at autopsy. However, new methods now allow physicians to identify patients with Alzheimer's disease with approximately 90 percent accuracy.

Using cultures of skin cells from Alzheimer's patients, Dr. René Etcheberrigaray of the National Institute of Neurological Disorders and Stroke and colleagues have found that a particular channel molecule that allows potassium to move in and out of cells is lacking or nonfunctional in Alzheimer's patients. This is significant because potassium plays an important role in memory formation. Researchers are hopeful that a skin test based on these new findings can be developed to allow easy diagnosis of the disease.

Investigators have determined that Alzheimer's disease causes the greatest deterioration in the basal forebrain, an area important for learning, memory, and other cognitive functions. Drs. Donald Price, Joseph Coyle, and Mahlon DeLong of Johns Hopkins University found that compared to age-matched control individuals, Alzheimer sufferers undergo a selective degeneration of 75 percent of the neurons in this region that produce the neurotransmitter acetylcholine. Studying the same region, Dr. Dominique Toran-Allerand and coworkers found receptors for estrogen and nerve growth factor. They believe that estrogen and nerve growth factor may regulate specific genes that influence survival, differentiation, regeneration, and plasticity of the neurons. In other words, just as estrogen turns specific genes on and off in other tissues like the uterine lining, it along with nerve growth factor and possibly other biologically active molecules may regulate specific genes in the cells affected by Alzheimer's disease.

Deficient estrogen levels are tied to Alzheimer's by other types of research. Dr. Victoria Luine, working with Dr. Bruce McEwen of Rockefeller University, has shown that a region of the rat brain that is comparable to the basal forebrain of humans may deteriorate after rat ovaries are removed. When Dr. Luine treats the deficient animals with estrogen, the deteriorated portion of the brain seems to be restored. While these data are from animals, they relate to one of the first observations concerning the effects of estrogen on cognitive function in postmenopausal women.

Dr. Herman Kantor and his colleagues in Dallas, Texas, made some remarkable observations when they studied postmenopausal women in a nursing home. The women were divided into two groups and tested to measure their psychological functioning. Women in one group were given estrogen therapy, but those in the other group received a placebo. After three months, the investigators noted a significant difference between the test results of the two groups. The differences were even more pronounced after three years of therapy when tests indicated that the estrogen-treated group had maintained their psychological functioning without deterioration but the psychological functioning of the placebo-treated group had declined considerably.

These observations parallel more recent evidence gathered at the Rockefeller University Hospital and Outpatient Clinic where researchers specifically looked for a connection between Alzheimer's disease and estrogen. They found that postmenopausal women with Alzheimer's disease had significantly lower levels of estrogen in their blood than normal women who were age- and weight-matched. The study was carried one step farther by administering oral estrogen replacement therapy to eight postmenopausal women diagnosed with Alzheimer's. Within six weeks, half the women demonstrated improved cognitive and emotional functioning as measured by standardized tests. The women who responded tended to be older and therefore would have had a more prolonged estrogen deficiency. It is interesting to note that these women also tended to have osteoporosis. Evidence supporting a relationship between estrogen replacement therapy and a decreased risk for Alzheimer's disease continues to mount. A recent study from the University of Southern California Medical School found that women who had used estrogen were 40 percent less likely to have Alzheimer's than women who had not. The decrease in risk appears to be dose related, so women who had taken higher doses of estrogen over a longer period of time had the lowest incidence of Alzheimer's. Related data from animals indicates that estrogen also helps maintain nerve growth factor and the number and function of neurons in the basal forebrain after the removal of both ovaries. Though researchers recognize the need for more prolonged investigation to determine the effectiveness and safety of estrogen replacement therapy before it can be considered for general therapeutic use, much preliminary data point to estrogen as a participant in the course of Alzheimer's disease. Continued research in this area is critical, since experts in neurobiology believe that dementia of the Alzheimer's type is reaching epidemic proportions.

4

More
Changes

---•---

Setting the Change in Motion

As a woman nears menopause, declining estrogen levels can cause irregular menstrual periods, hot flashes, "crawly skin," visual problems, migraines, hair loss, moustache growth, incontinence, as well as a number of other peculiar physical symptoms. What causes estrogen to support so many of a woman's body functions for 30 or 40 years and then leave them in the lurch? One controversial proposal posits that women are living far in excess of the number of years that nature intended and are thus outliving their reproductive potential. The physiological data have not yet been completely untangled, but certain facts are known. For one thing, it is true that the ovaries "run out" of the 400,000 egg-containing primary follicles that a young woman has at puberty. These are limited in number at birth with no possibility of additional follicles ever being formed. Throughout the reproductive years, the follicles serve as the body's estrogen and progesterone factories, but at each menstrual cycle, anywhere from 10 to 1000 of the primary follicles are lost to ovulation and degeneration. By the beginning of the climacteric, usually in the late 30s to mid 40s, only about 10,000 primary follicles remain interspersed in the cells and fibrous tissue of the ovary, and the number continues to decline.

By menopause, the surfaces of the ovaries are scarred and pitted at more than 400 sites where ovulation has occurred. Each ovary has shrunk to about one-third the size it was in the woman's 40s, few if any egg-containing follicles remain, and the postmenopausal ovary has lost the ability to manufacture estrogen and progesterone. Some argue that it is as if the ovary has a built-in clock that runs down as the number of primary follicles disappear, thus setting a limit on the estrogen-rich reproductive years.

Other experts believe that the reproduction control center, the part of the brain that prompts each repetitive menstrual cycle and regulates the fluctuating hormone cycles, is also instrumental in initiating menopause. Dr. Terry Parkening at the University of Texas Medical Branch at Galveston presents strong evidence that supports this proposal. He removed the ovaries of young mice and replaced them with ovaries from mice too old to any longer reproduce. The young mice were able to mate and have babies using the old ovaries. The investigators speculate that the old mouse brain was no longer capable of stimulating the ovaries to function, but that the young mouse brain was able to provide the correct hormonal cues. Their argument is reinforced by additional data. When the ovaries of old animals that could no longer reproduce were removed and replaced with ovaries from young mice, the old animals were still *unable* to reproduce. This strengthens the suggestion that the old mouse brain simply could not provide the proper cues to set the reproductive process in motion. This evidence supporting brain-initiated menopause is certainly persuasive although not conclusive.

Hormone supplies are significantly reduced regardless of where menopause is initiated. Ovulation no longer occurs so there is no corpus luteum to produce progesterone or inhibin. However, the female body is not left completely lacking in hormones. According to Dr. Morris Notelovitz, coauthor of *Estrogen: Yes or No?*, the ovaries continue to produce small amounts of estradiol after menopause. The postmenopausal ovaries, as well as the cortex of the adrenal gland, continue to produce another steroid hormone, *androstenedione*, that is transported to other body sites, primarily adipose or fatty tissue, where it is converted into estrogen. This conversion process continues to become more efficient as a woman ages and provides basically all the estrogen after menopause. *Estradiol*, the primary estrogen of the reproductive years, is in short supply, however, since it is produced only sparingly by conversion from androstenedione. *Estrone*, another estrogen, that is only about one-third as active as estradiol, is produced in larger quantities and becomes the principal estrogen in the years after menopause. The following chart indicates the low levels of estradiol in postmenopausal women. The decrease is particularly obvious when postmenopausal levels of estradiol are compared to the changing levels of the hormone that are normal during the reproductive years. Notice that adult males also produce a small amounts of estradiol.

Adult Females		pg/mL Estradiol
Follicular Phase	− 12 Days	10–50
	− 4 Days	60–200
Ovulation	0 Days	120–375
Luteal Phase	+ 2 Days	50–155
	+ 6 Days	60–260
	+ 12 Days	15–115
Postmenopausal		0–14
Adult Males		6–44

The overall deficit of estradiol after menopause provokes changes in several body tissues and delivers a message that is no doubt confusing to the hypothalamus.

Mixed Messages in the Hypothalamus

Estrogen, like other hormones, can convey different messages by virtue of the amount present. The brain, especially the hypothalamus, continuously monitors levels of estrogen in the bloodstream and responds to changes. For example, at the beginning of the menstrual cycle, *low levels of estrogen* signal estrogen receptors in the hypothalamus to *stimulate increased release of FSH and LH* from the pituitary. These gonadotropins travel to the ovaries and set them in motion. Ovarian follicle cells are prompted to produce more estrogen and the menstrual cycle is underway. Near midcycle, the follicle cells are at the peak of estrogen production. This is reflected in *high levels of estrogen* in the bloodstream that notify estrogen receptors in the hypothalamus to *reduce the release of FSH* from the pituitary because estrogen levels are sufficient to carry on menstrual-cycle functions.

During the climacteric, the hypothalamus interprets the declining level of estrogen as a persistent message to send more FSH and LH to the ovaries. It secretes gonadotropin-releasing hormone that urges the pituitary to release FSH and LH in an attempt to jar the ovaries into action. However, the few remaining follicle cells are less responsive to FSH and LH, and are unable to secrete enough estrogen to satisfy the "expectations" of the estrogen receptors in the brain. As menopause approaches, the very elaborate communication systems of the body have no built-in mechanism to tell the brain that the lifetime supply of eggs and follicles has been exhausted. Menstrual cycles are no longer necessary or even possible.

In an attempt to initiate a new menstrual cycle, FSH levels soar and average 18 times more than the highest amounts normally reached in the reproductive years. LH production also escalates and exceeds the levels of reproductive years by 3 times. It is clear that the hypothalamus and pituitary still have the ability to respond to estrogen, since FSH and LH levels decrease to those typical of the reproductive years if a woman is given estrogen replacement therapy. In an untreated woman, circulating levels of FSH and LH remain high for years to come.

FSH – A Harbinger of Menopause

Rising FSH levels are so characteristic of the perimenopause that physicians commonly monitor them for signs of change as a woman approaches menopause. The following table lists the "normal" reproductive ranges of FSH and LH, as well as the hormone levels that are usually observed near and after menopause. For comparison, the chart includes normal levels of FSH and LH for women taking oral contraceptives, women who are pregnant, and males. (Yes, males have FSH and LH. In them, the hormones stimulate sperm and testosterone production.)

Adult Females		MIU/mL FSH	MIU/mL LH
Follicular phase	1–14 days	1.5–6.3	2.8–15.2
Peak phase	15–17 days	3.9–23.4	12.1–66.0
Luteal phase	18–28 days	1.1–3.4	2.6–11.7
Postmenopausal		25.2–100.0	22.0–78.0
Oral contraceptive		1.2–3.6	3.0–9.9
Pregnancy		0.0–4.0	25.0–100.0
Adult Males		1.3–6.3	4.0–12.6

The levels of FSH in postmenopausal women exceed those ever reached during a normal menstrual cycle. Even during the brief peak phase of the menstrual cycle (near ovulation), FSH levels are below those present in postmenopausal women. The postmenopausal rise in LH levels is distinct but not as substantial as the increase in FSH. It is helpful to keep an accurate account of the first day of each menstrual cycle so test results can be interpreted in the proper portion of the cycle. It is also important to remember that hormone tests are not always a total answer. According to Dr. Wulf Utian, coauthor of *Managing Your Menopause*, subtle hormone changes that are within the "normal limits" may still provoke menopause symptoms in some women. The table should serve only as a reference for discussing individual test results with your physician.

It is perfectly acceptable to ask your physician for a copy of your test results. A doctor may assume that a woman will not understand the results or that her only concern is whether test results are good or bad. Being told that "Your test results are fine" may be reassuring, but knowing the results and asking questions allows a woman to understand what is happening inside her body. It makes her a participant and not a bystander in her menopause passage, and most physicians welcome a woman who takes interest and accepts responsibility for her own health care.

Irregular Menstrual Periods – An Early Sign

Rising FSH levels are an excellent clinical indicator of impending menopause. Irregular menstrual periods are often another early sign that the body is changing. Irregular periods may begin in a woman's late 30s or early 40s, sometimes preceding menopause by so many years that the link with fluctuating hormone levels and eventual menopause is not obvious. There seems to be no definite set of changes in menstrual cycles that relate to the climacteric or perimenopause years.

Generally the decreasing levels of estadiol result in a gradual shortening of the luteal phase or second portion of the menstrual cycle. This is followed by a decrease in progesterone that can promote an increase in the overall length of the menstrual cycle. Although some women experience a decrease in menstrual flow, others, probably the majority, encounter a heavier menstrual flow that sometimes includes blood clots. Blood clots are present as the endometrium is sloughed, but in normal menstrual bleeding natural enzymes have time to act on the clots and break them down before they leave the body as part of the menstrual flow. When the menstrual flow is very brisk, the enzymes apparently do not have sufficient time to break up the clots before they are discharged.

In the years preceding menopause, a woman should not be alarmed by irregular menstrual periods since they are often an early sign of normal hormonal changes. In the majority of cases, they are due to some abnormality in the hormonal balance between the hypothalamus, pituitary, and ovaries. However, persistent heavy or otherwise irregular menstrual periods can also be a symptom of polyps, fibroids, or some other condition unrelated to menopause and should definitely be discussed with a physician.

In some cases, sorting out the cause of menstrual irregularities may require a *dilatation* and *curettage* or "*D & C*" (sometimes also referred to as a "Dusting and Cleaning"). Currently, almost one million D&Cs are performed each year in the United States. The procedure requires that the patient receive general anesthesia. Then the cervix is *dilated* or stretched to allow easy access to the uterine lining, which is *curetted* or scraped off. A D&C does carry some risk because a general anesthesia is administered. There are also occasional complications that include perforation of the wall of the uterus, excessive bleeding, infection, or scarring of the uterine lining.

Many D&Cs are necessary procedures to determine the cause of abnormal bleeding, but some are considered questionable by physicians like Dr. Herbert Keyser, author of *Women Under the Knife*. Dr. Keyser and others believe that an endometrial biopsy, which obtains only a small sample of the uterine lining for analysis, carries less risk and can often identify the cause of irregular bleeding. In a type of biopsy known as an endometrial aspiration, or a "mini D&C," a small tube is inserted through the cervix, and a sample of the uterine lining is removed by suction. This simpler procedure presents a much lower risk of complications since it is performed under local anesthesia, does not require stretching of the cervix, and involves fewer instruments being inserted into the uterus. It also entails considerably less expense, and, in some cases, is sufficient for the doctor to diagnose and treat a problem. In others, the endometrial biopsy confirms that a D&C is indeed warranted.

Irregular periods are the hallmark of approaching menopause for many women and a signal to be alert for other changes. However, a great many women have regular menstrual periods up to and including the very last one, menopause. With no advance warning that menopause is on its way, it is sometimes difficult for these women to recognize other menopause-related symptoms.

Hot Flashes and Other Peculiar Sensations

Approximately 85 percent of all women will experience *hot flashes* during the climacteric. The hot flash, probably the most notorious sign of menopause, is one of a group of temporary but quite peculiar sensations that include night sweats, sleep disturbances, insomnia, irritability, forgetfulness, dizziness, headache, migraine, visual disturbances, dry eyes, nausea, and paresthesia (sensations like pins and needles or insects crawling on your skin). This odd assortment of changes scarcely seems to have a common thread to tie them together or connect them to changes occurring in the reproductive system. Yet, most of these strange symptoms are thought to be related to *vasomotor instability* (inconsistency of the mechanisms that regulate the size of blood vessels) that is directly or indirectly caused by factors associated with decreasing levels of estrogen in the bloodstream. Hot flashes are the best studied example of this group of symptoms.

A hot flash episode starts as a warm sensation in the neck and quickly spreads to the face and upper body. The unexpected rise in temperature is usually, but not always, accompanied by perspiration and sometimes by other symptoms like palpitations (rapid heart rate), headache, nausea, and dizziness. Many women describe a sort of premonition or a funny feeling that immediately precedes the rise in temperature. Researchers term the funny feeling a *hot flash* and the actual rise in temperature a *hot flush*, but hot flash remains the term most women and many physicians commonly use to describe the entire event. Once begun, a complete hot flash episode usually lasts 3 to 6 minutes, although it may extend up to an hour. These unpredictable events can strike singly, but sometimes they come in multiples of 30, 40, or even 50 either in rapid succession or sporadically spaced through the course of a day. About 50 percent of the women who do have hot flashes find that they persist for about one year. Another 30 percent experience hot flashes for about 2.5 years; 20 percent of hot flash sufferers endure the unpleasant episodes for 5 to 10 years. A small number of women—maybe 2 to 3 percent—continue to have hot flashes for life.

Body weight can indirectly influence the number and frequency of hot flashes. On average, overweight women have fewer hot flashes than thin women. This makes good sense if you remember that after menopause the adipose tissue serves as the major site of conversion of androgen (from the ovaries and adrenal glands) to estrogen. This gives overweight women with more abundant adipose tissue a physiological edge that provides them an added degree of protection from hot flashes. Unnecessary pounds, however, go hand in hand with an increased risk of cardiovascular disease that can be much more devastating than hot flashes.

Declining estrogen certainly plays a role in triggering hot flashes, but it is not the sole cause of these episodes. The *temperature-regulating* center in the hypothalamus of the brain and the neurotransmitter, *norepinephrine*, that it releases also appear to be involved when a hot flash occurs. Scientists speculate that when the body overheats under normal conditions, the temperature-regulating center releases norepinephrine that sets in motion mechanisms promoting natural heat loss. For example, blood vessels near the skin dilate (enlarge) and permit heat to dissipate from the body's surface. Perspiration, another consequence of overheating, cools the body as it evaporates from the skin. How does estrogen fit into this picture? Estrogen regulates the receptors that control the release of norepinephrine. Researchers speculate that during menopause low estrogen levels reduce the number of receptors that control norepinephrine release; this causes the temperature-regulating cells to fire abnormally and release norepinephrine at inappropriate times. The norepinephrine creates the illusion that the body is overheated and triggers normal heat-loss mechanisms in an attempt to end the imaginary spell of overheating created by incorrect information in the hypothalamus.

Dr. Robert Freedman of Wayne State University in Detroit heads a research team that used two drugs to test the hypothesis that norepinephrine is indeed involved in triggering hot flashes. Both drugs work by affecting special nerve cell receptors in the hypothalamus that regulate whether or not norepinephrine is released. One drug, *yohimbine, stimulates* the receptors and boosts norepinephrine levels. The other drug, *clonidine, subdues* the receptors and inhibits norepinephrine release. The effects of the drugs were compared on a symptomatic group of 9 postmenopausal women known to have 6 to 12 hot flashes per day. During the experiment, the women were hooked to a continuous intravenous drip of saline solution and were not told when either drug was added. When yohimbine was added to the saline, it triggered hot flashes in these women. The addition of clonidine decreased the number of hot flashes they experienced. Dr.

Freedman and his colleagues believe this indicates that norepinephrine plays a major role in triggering hot flashes.

It is important to note that neither yohimbine nor clonidine affected another group of 6 postmenopausal women who had never experienced hot flashes. These women represent that fortunate 15 percent of all women who do not have hot flashes. Scientists speculate that women who never or seldom experience hot flashes may have some special trait that compensates for the loss of estrogen. Perhaps these women have more abundant norepinephrine-regulating receptors or some other unique characteristic that spares them from hot flashes.

Experiments like those performed by Dr. Freedman continue to add more pieces to the puzzle of hot flashes and also contribute information about drugs that suppress hot flashes. Clonidine and another drug, lofexidine, subdue the release of norepinephrine by acting on the receptors in the temperature-regulating cells of the hypothalamus. Both reduce hot flashes, but neither is as effective as estradiol in the management of hot flashes. They do, however, provide alternate drug choices for women who cannot take estrogen.

Nausea, another annoying result of the hormone changes of the climacteric, sometimes accompanies hot flashes or may appear separately. The precise hormone activity that causes menopause-related nausea is not clear, but it may be somewhat similar to the cause of morning sickness. Hot flashes and nausea are well-known signs of menopause, but they can still be mistaken for symptoms of some other unrelated illness. Sandra was only 44 years old when she first experienced unexplained waves of nausea while working with her horses. She had two or three occurrences sporadically spaced over a three-month period. During each episode, the nausea was accompanied by hyperventilation, diarrhea, and fatigue. Sandra also got very hot and flushed but attributed that to the fact that she was working outside. She thought the incidents were caused by her chronic thyroid condition or possibly some heat-related illness. It is easy to miss the relationship of symptoms like these and menopause. This is especially true for women in their late 30s or early 40s who like Sandra are still having relatively regular menstrual cycles. Sandra's physician, suspicious that the hot spells might be hot flashes, checked Sandra's thyroid hormones and also checked her FSH level. The thyroid was normal, but the FSH was elevated to a postmenopausal level of 40.1 MIU/mL. Sandra's hot spells were indeed hot flashes that were not accompanied by profuse perspiration. Sandra got quick relief from low-dose estrogen therapy and within two months was completely free of the nausea, fatigue, and hot flashes.

Is There a Bug on Me?

One of the most unusual of the climacteric complaints is *paresthesia*, a tingling sensation or the feeling that "something" is creeping on the skin, but the something isn't really there. A more familiar type of paresthesia is experienced following local anesthesia for dental work. It is the tingling, slightly numb, pins-and-needles response that occurs as the anesthesia wears off. During the climacteric, paresthesia can occur with no outside stimulus. In these cases, women usually say an episode of paresthesia makes them feel like insects are crawling over their skin. The sensation is real and a number of women do "feel" creatures crawling on them.

Just what prompts sensory nerves to fire and cause this creepy-crawly feeling on the skin isn't clear. There is no nerve damage. The sensation is a trick of the nervous system that is annoying but apparently harmless. However, repeated bouts of paresthesia should be discussed with a physician. These episodes also occur as a symptom of a peripheral neuropathy, a condition that does include nerve damage.

When You Can't See Straight

It is sometimes difficult to make the connection between a strange new symptom and the climacteric, especially if the new symptom is vision related. The eyes hardly seem closely linked with the reproductive system or the hormone ups and downs that precede menopause. Because of this ambiguous association, dry eyes and decreased visual acuity (sharpness of an object) may head the list of difficult-to-diagnose problems that can occur during the climacteric. Furthermore, they may affect a fairly large number of women.

A research team in Vienna recently studied a group of 1287 women who visited a physician with concerns related to the climacteric. Rarely did a woman complain of a problem with her eyes or her vision. However, when directly questioned by the physician, 35 percent of the women had an eye complaint that was found to be obviously associated with the onset of the climacteric. Strange as it may seem, the eye has estrogen receptors and relies on estrogen stimulation. When estrogen levels drop, the eyes can become dry and irritated and vision can become a little fuzzy. The Austrian research team determined that the decrease in visual acuity was most likely associated with insufficient lacrimal fluid (tears) and concluded that estrogen apparently affects the lacrimal glands and conjunctiva (the membrane covering the inside of the eyelids and the outside of the eyeballs). The problems were very responsive to estrogen once they were recognized as menopause-related symptoms. Most of the women in the study reported substantial improvement and/or almost complete relief from their symptoms following three months of hormone replacement therapy that included estrogen. Some authorities speculate that this obscure symptom of menopause may be related to the many cases of contact-lens intolerance that develop during the perimenopause.

It is unfortunate that many visual problems go undiagnosed because women do not report them to their physician along with other symptoms associated with the climacteric. A woman may be more inclined to relate visual difficulties to her ophthalmologist who does not specialize in problems of the climacteric and may fail to relate the visual problem with menopause. Women and physicians, including ophthalmologists, need to be made aware of this fairly common menopause symptom that often goes undiagnosed.

Migraines

Migraine headaches are another curious symptom of menopause that at first glance appear unrelated to the changing estrogen levels of the climacteric. However, women with a history of migraines are often plagued with more frequent episodes during the climacteric while others experience migraines for the first time during perimenopause or shortly after surgical menopause (hysterectomy with ovaries removed).

Estimates of the number of people who suffer from migraines annually range from 8 to 18 million people. A 1992 study in the *Journal of the American Medical Association* suggested that in the United States approximately 8.7 million women and 2.6 million men experience migraine headaches each year. Whatever the actual total number of migraine sufferers, there is no question that the majority of migraine patients are women. The reason for the disproportionate number of female sufferers is not clear, but it may be related to fluctuating hormone levels or sex-linked inheritance.

For a long time, physicians believed that migraines were precipitated by changes in blood-vessel diameter that altered the pattern of blood flow to the brain. These alterations do occur, but migraines are now thought to be a consequence of an imbalance in the amount of certain neurochemicals, especially *serotonin*, a neurotransmitter that normally plays a role in pain perception and mood changes.

There is no cure for migraines but there are several drug treatments in use or being tested for use that include analgesics, nonsteroidal anti-inflammatory drugs, ergotamines, serotonin agonists, dopamine agonists, adrenergic beta antagonists (beta-blockers), and calcium channel blockers. These are aimed at alleviating pain and preventing future migraines. Which drug is prescribed depends on many factors including the intensity and duration of the migraine and the patient's ability to tolerate different drugs and drug combinations. Some of the most useful treatments may work by regulating the size of blood vessels, although it is not clearly established that vasoconstriction is an effective therapy. *Sumatriptan* (*Imitrex*), an injectable serotonin agonist, was developed especially to treat migraine and is an effective treatment for some. It works by stimulating particular serotonin receptors that are thought to cause constriction of blood vessels in the head. The bottom line is that there is no cure for migraines and available drugs to alleviate pain and prevent future attacks work for some and not for others.

Migraine headaches are classified as *common migraines* or *classic migraines*. Common migraines manifest as severe, throbbing pain on one side of the head and can be accompanied by nausea, vomiting, cold hands, dizziness, and/or sensitivity to light and noise. A woman may experience mood changes including irritability, excitability, depression, or euphoria hours or even days before the actual headache strikes. A classic migraine is similar to a common migraine except that it lacks the preheadache mood changes. Instead, these headaches are preceded by an *aura* or change in visual and/or sensory perception that usually materializes about one-half hour before the headache pain begins. An aura may manifest as flashing lights or dark spots before the eyes, loss of half the field of vision in one or both eyes, light-headedness, difficulty concentrating, or confusion. Some migraine patients experience a visual aura without the pain of a migraine headache. This phenomenon is referred to as an *ophthalmic migraine.*

Common and classic migraines and probably ophthalmic migraines can be set off by a number of stimuli including chocolate, peanuts, aged cheese, red wine, monosodium glutamate (MSG), bright flashing lights, or changes in blood sugar or hormone levels. Classic migraines can also be prompted by visual triggers like staring at linear patterns in striped wallpaper or blinds. In other cases, there is no apparent trigger that initiates a migraine.

Research in this area is scant. The only real consensus is that migraine headaches and/or ophthalmic migraines that occur during puberty or menopause are probably related to unstable estrogen levels since they seem to occur more frequently when the body is establishing a new level of estrogen production—increased during puberty and decreased during the climacteric or following surgical menopause. The direction of change may not be as critical as the state of flux to which the body is adjusting. Not enough data are available to explain what causes menopause-related migraines, but I have my own story to relate and my own hypothesis to offer.

Like many women in the years of perimenopause, I had never had a migraine or any unusual vision problems. I was understandably distressed when the center of the visual field of my left eye periodically became very dim. Not realizing that this unusual symptom might be related to menopause, I went to see my ophthalmologist. He found no anatomical abnormality, and referred me to my family physician for a series of blood tests that eliminated possible causes like a thyroid disorder. I was then referred to a neurologist for further tests. In his referral letter, the ophthalmologist alluded to ophthalmic migraine as a possible diagnosis although it was not one that had come immediately to his mind. The neurologist agreed that ophthalmic migraine was a strong possibility.

Unfortunately, there is no diagnostic test for any type of migraine. A diagnosis is reached only by ruling out all other possibilities. A test called a carotid doppler determined that blood flow to my head was normal and a cranial MRI (magnetic resonance imaging) ruled out the presence of tumors. These results made the diagnosis of ophthalmic migraine fairly definite. As mentioned above, treatment for migraine offers limited choices. To add to the difficulty, drugs commonly used to treat migraine headaches have apparently not been rigorously tested for their effectiveness in treating ophthalmic migraine.

A group of drugs known as *β-blockers* that are commonly used in patients with cardiovascular disease are sometimes also used in an attempt to prevent migraines. I took a moderately low-dose β-blocker for about two months. It may have caused a marginal improvement in my vision but certainly not a clear-cut change. The drug did cause incredible fatigue that rendered me about one level of consciousness above a sleepwalker. The minimal improvement was just not worth compromising a reasonable quality of life, so I discontinued taking the β-blocker although no other therapeutic alternatives were offered.

The neurologist was unaware of any studies that had evaluated the use of estrogen replacement therapy in the management of migraines or ophthalmic migraines even though the symptoms are often related to the climacteric. I reasoned, however, that since the ophthalmic migraines are sometimes associated with fluctuating levels of estrogen, a stable base level of estrogen induced by estrogen replacement therapy might be a logical course of treatment. After all, other transient symptoms of menopause like hot flashes and nausea also occur when estrogen production is readjusting to a new level. These and many other symptoms of menopause disappear with time or with estrogen replacement therapy. Estrogen therapy might not eliminate ophthalmic migraines, but, then again, maybe it would.

My physician checked my hormone levels, which had indeed shifted to postmenopausal levels even though my periods were still quite regular. This made estrogen replacement therapy a sound course of action even without the consideration of ophthalmic migraines. Within the first month of estrogen replacement therapy, I noted a marked reduction in the number and intensity of the visual aberrations. Within two months, the ophthalmic migraines had completely disappeared. This provides no scientific proof that estrogen replacement therapy cured my ophthalmic migraines. I was an experimental "group of one," with no control group, which is not an acceptable experimental design. However, the ophthalmic migraines had persisted and increased in frequency and intensity for over a year prior to the estrogen therapy. Their disappearance with the initiation of estrogen replacement therapy may have been a coincidence—then again, maybe not. The cause of ophthalmic migraines and migraine headaches and the efficacy of using estrogen as a treatment in menopausal women with these conditions are areas that await proper scientific investigation. In the interim, some researchers are investigating other unique therapies for migraine.

Dr. James Couch, a neurologist at Southern Illinois University School of Medicine, encourages sex for the relief of migraines. Of 52 migraine sufferers (not necessarily in perimenopause) who made love during migraine episodes, 8 reported that their headaches disappeared and 16 experienced relief from the headache pain. Dr. Couch believes that sex could also be helpful in easing tension-headache pain. Research in this area has just begun, but information concerning relief from migraine is so scarce that sex is certainly worth a try.

Hair-Raising Changes

Another set of menopause symptoms collectively called *somatic changes* or body changes are very different from the symptoms caused by vasomotor instability. Somatic changes include wrinkles, loss of muscle tone, hirsutism, and thinning scalp hair. As strange as it may seem, these too are a result of changing levels of steroid hormones. Wrinkles and loss of muscle tone occur as a natural part of the aging process but are accentuated by declining levels of estrogen. Diminishing estrogen levels can result in drier skin that promotes wrinkles but is not their sole cause. Similarly, a reduction in estrogen tends to hasten the loss of muscle tone especially in those who lead fairly sedentary lives. Estrogen replacement therapy does encourage supple skin, although it will not eliminate wrinkles or restore lost muscle. Declining estrogen even changes the distribution of fat stores in the female figure and the "waist" may disappear. Exercise is especially critical to maintain muscle tone and stay in shape as estrogen levels fall.

Hirsutism and balding are not experienced by all women. When they do occur, they are encouraged by testosterone that is present throughout the reproductive and postreproductive phases of life. In the reproductive years, abundant estrogen supplies "override" the influences of testosterone that would otherwise promote characteristics like facial hair and coarse body hair. However, the tables can turn during the climacteric and postmenopausal years. Testosterone production does not increase—as a matter of fact, it drops slightly—but estrogen levels drop even more and may become too low to "overpower" testosterone's influence on the receptors that control hair texture and growth. When this occurs, testosterone can transform previously light, fine upper-lip hair into a moustache. Similarly, body hair on arms, legs, and chest may change in appearance and texture and become dark and coarse. Scalp hair, on the other hand, may become sparse when testosterone is unopposed by adequate estrogen supplies. Estrogen replacement therapy is usually very effective in counteracting coarse facial and body hair. Estrogen's ability to reverse these changes surely added support to the claims of physicians in the 1960s who hailed estrogen as a virtual fountain of youth that maintained the femininity of women nearing menopause.

More About Menopause and Sex

Declining estrogen levels also have a consequence on all the reproductive tissues and organs. Changes in the breast tissue are often pronounced during the climacteric. The abundant estrogen of the reproductive years fosters the development of breasts and keeps them firm with milk glands ever ready for pregnancy and childbirth. As menopause approaches, diminishing estrogen levels are no longer sufficient to prod the milk glands to remain available for use. The milk glands shrivel, and breasts lose their firmness and begin to droop. The sag of the breast is usually emphasized by the loss of elasticity in Cooper's ligament, a band of tissue that serves as a support system for the breast tissue. Obese women with large breasts may be especially affected by these changes, while women with small breasts may find them even smaller and flatter after menopause. Other women experience an increase in fatty tissue in the breast area that leaves breast size similar to what it was before menopause.

Other external reproductive structures also undergo obvious changes due to decreasing estrogen stimulation. The pubic hair covering the mons (the rounded, fatty prominence over the pubic bone) becomes thin and scant. Fat and other tissues underlying the labia major (outer folds of skin) and labia minor (inner folds of mucosa) that surround the openings to the urethra and vagina atrophy.

Internal reproductive structures are not spared as the estrogen supply fades. The shrinking ovaries have already been mentioned. The uterus, no longer on standby for pregnancy, shrivels until it is about one-fourth its former size. The uterine walls become thinner and cease normal functions. After menopause, the cervix also diminishes in size and loses much of its ability to secrete prostaglandins. There are no studies that indicate what effect, if any, decreased amounts of prostaglandins have on the body after menopause. Like the rest of the internal reproductive structures, the Fallopian tubes also shrivel, and their inner lining loses most of the cilia. Scientists have found that the presence of cilia in the Fallopian tubes is yet another estrogen-dependent characteristic. The cilia simply cannot survive without sufficient estrogen stimulation.

Shriveling of the ovaries, uterus, cervix, and Fallopian tubes may never be perceived by a woman, but vaginal atrophy (shrinking of the vagina) can seriously affect sexual activity as estrogen levels drop. As the estrogen supply dwindles, the vagina loses much of its elasticity, the walls become significantly thinner, and the entire structure narrows and shortens. In addition, the glands that produce lubricating secretions during sexual arousal shrink and virtually shut down. The postmenopausal vagina is very fragile and dry. These very real physical changes can make intercourse uncomfortable or even painful. Vaginal atrophy can occur any time during the perimenopause but often becomes noticeable within the 6-month period following menopause (especially following surgical menopause). However, the course of atrophy is variable and can progress more slowly. A few women do not experience uncomfortable sex for 5 or sometimes 10 years after menopause.

As previously mentioned, vaginal atrophy may have kindled the myth that menopausal women lose interest in sex. The more likely reality is that postmenopausal women have little interest in painful intercourse. Today this need not be a problem because vaginal atrophy can be readily corrected. Symptoms can sometimes be alleviated with a lubricant. Oil-based substances promote vaginal infections and should be avoided, but a number of water-soluble products like K-Y Jelly are available and can be used just prior to intercourse. Replens is a relatively new water-soluble product that can be applied well in advance of intercourse. It has long-lasting effects that promote the lubrication of vaginal tissues for two or three days.

Estrogen-containing creams do much more than provide artificial lubrication, but these are available only by prescription. Vaginal tissues absorb the estrogen, and the atrophy begins to reverse rapidly. However, it is sometimes a matter of weeks before the maximum benefits of the estrogen cream are realized. Vaginal wall tissues grow thicker and less fragile, and the lubricating glands of the vagina are rejuvenated and begin to secrete natural lubricants. Vaginal tissues may never have the same resilience and lubrication capabilities as they had in the reproductive years, but the changes are wonderful and should greatly enhance the pleasure of intercourse. A healthy sex life can require a little physical maintenance, but intercourse should be as comfortable and pleasurable after menopause as it was before.

Incontinence

The urinary tract is another system that can be upset by decreased levels of estrogen. Scientists have recently determined that estrogen receptors are present in the bladder, the urethra (the tube that empties the bladder), and the connective tissue surrounding the urethra. It is not surprising that decreasing estrogen levels of the climacteric can trigger a number of atrophic changes in these urinary tract tissues and promote recurrent infections or other medical problems.

Incontinence, the involuntary loss of urine, is one of the most troublesome consequences of urinary tract decline. Not every postmenopausal woman suffers from incontinence, but the considerable number of television and magazine advertisements promoting an assortment of pads and "adult diapers" serves as an indicator of the prevalence of the problem. Current studies confirm that incontinence is probably more widespread than previously realized.

The exact number of postmenopausal women troubled with incontinence is not clear, but the total number of people who suffer from incontinence from all causes is large. The U.S. Department of Health and Human Services estimates that urinary incontinence (due to all causes) affects at least 10 million men and women in the United States. The problem is especially common among people 65 years and older. Incontinence affects 15 to 30 percent of nonhospitalized people in this age group where it is more common in women than men and more prevalent in white women than black.

"Officially" there are discrepancies in the number of postmenopausal women reported to suffer from incontinence related to the climacteric. Some researchers indicate that as few as 17 percent of the postmenopausal women surveyed experience incontinence while other investigators report that as many as 50 percent of postmenopausal women are incontinent. Different sampling techniques used by the various investigators are at least partially responsible for the wide range of values. A careful study using current sampling techniques was recently performed by a group from the Netherlands. They reported that incontinence was present in approximately 26 percent of the postmenopausal women they surveyed. About 7 percent of the women suffered from incontinence on a daily basis and the remainder experienced incontinence at a lower frequency. Still, the postmenopausal women in the study group experienced incontinence more than twice as often as they had before menopause.

Unfortunately, few women seek medical attention for problems of incontinence and so many suffer unnecessarily. Estrogen replacement therapy can make a big difference in the lives of postmenopausal women troubled with incontinence. In addition to estrogen replacement therapy, special exercises termed *Kegel exercises* can be done on a daily basis to strengthen the muscles that control urine retention. Some physicians recommend practicing Kegel exercises by contracting muscles to stop urination midstream. This maneuver uses the same muscles required for Kegel exercises. Once a woman knows which muscles to use, Kegel exercises can be done almost anywhere. The exercises require tightening the pelvic muscles and holding the muscle contraction for ten seconds. Three sets of ten repetitions performed daily are sufficient to give many women increased bladder control.

While Kegel exercises improve bladder control, doctors from the University of Michigan recently reported that some other forms of exercise may promote incontinence in later life. John DeLancey and colleagues surveyed 326 women who ranged in age from 17 to 68 years (average age 38.5). The researchers were particularly interested in the effects of running and high impact aerobics on the urinary tract. They found that 38 percent of the women who were runners and 36 percent of the women who did high-impact aerobic workouts sometimes lost bladder control during exercise. Childbearing seems to have a definite influence on exercise-related incontinence since the problem was more common among women who had three vaginal deliveries than among women with no children. Running and aerobics both involve a lot of bouncing up and down that apparently stresses the bladder. Dr. DeLancey recommends daily Kegel exercises to strengthen pelvic muscles and emptying the bladder before running or aerobic workouts. He suggests that a persistent problem might be improved by trying a "more bladder friendly" form of exercise like swimming or bicycling and emphasizes that women should not give up on exercise—it has too many positive benefits.

Urinary Tract Infections

Experts estimate that 10 to 15 percent of women over 60 years of age have frequent urinary tract infections that represent a significant health problem. Premenopausal women are protected from similar urinary tract infections by higher levels of circulating estrogen. The presence of estrogen in the vaginal area encourages the growth of a particular type of bacteria, *lactobacilli*, that helps keep the urinary tract healthy. The metabolic activity of lactobacilli produces *lactic acid*. This substance maintains the vagina at a low pH that inhibits the growth of many pathogenic or disease-causing bacteria. Some lactobacilli also produce hydrogen peroxide that is thought to be an additional deterrent to the growth of harmful bacteria. As estrogen levels fall during the climacteric, the lactobacilli disappear from the vagina and the pH rises. This makes conditions favorable for the growth of other organisms, especially *Escherichia coli*, which is the predominant form of vaginal bacteria present in postmenopausal women. *Escherichia coli* promote vaginal infections that can be treated with antibiotics but tend to recur with some regularity. Prevention of the infections is a more desirable therapy. Studies now indicate that estrogen replacement therapy reduces recurrent urinary tract infections (see Chapter 8).

There is one additional note on the topic of urinary tract infections. Evidence exists that vaginal tissue dryness is conducive to infection. Dr. June Reinisch, former director of The Kinsey Institute at Indiana University, reports that postmenopausal women who regularly orgasm may have a reduced chance of contracting urinary tract or vaginal infections. She believes that regular sexual activity provides continuous lubrication of the vaginal area and counteracts dryness, therefore reducing the likelihood of infection. Regular sexual activity is not a cure all. However, it is interesting that accumulating evidence indicates sex may have some therapeutic value for a number of menopause symptoms.

5

Menopause
Before Your
Time

Young Women Facing Menopause

Lynn and her husband, Jake, had put off having a family so Lynn could get her career on solid ground. By the time she turned 30, they were anxious to have their first child. Instead of signs of pregnancy, Lynn was startled by irregular menstrual periods, hot flashes, night sweats, and nausea. The symptoms were those expected at menopause, but Lynn was much too young for that—or was she? With great concern, she described the peculiar changes to her physician. A Pap smear, pelvic exam, and a number of tests revealed no unusual findings. Lynn was astonished, however, to hear the physician explain that *her FSH levels were well within the range normally found in a postmenopausal woman.* Lynn is one of a number of young women who reach menopause long before the average age of 51 years. They are robbed of the anticipated number of reproductive years, as well as several years of natural estrogen that protect against bone loss and cardiovascular disease. Premature menopause is most commonly diagnosed in women aged 35 to 40, but women in their 20s and early 30s can also find themselves past menopause.

Doctors do not know why menopause comes so early for some women. Heredity may play a role since premature menopause also occurs among the mothers and sisters of 13 percent of the women who experience an early end to their reproductive years. Other authorities speculate that premature menopause is caused by an autoimmune reaction. If this is true, the body sees its own follicles as foreign invaders akin to interloping bacteria or viruses. No longer recognized as the body's own tissue, the irreplaceable follicles and the immature eggs they contain are attacked and destroyed. If premature menopause is indeed an autoimmune disease, it would not be a unique condition. Rheumatoid arthritis, multiple sclerosis, myasthenia gravis, and lupus erythematosus are other all-too-familiar forms of autoimmune diseases.

With special medical help, some women have been able to become pregnant after premature menopause. Dr. Jerome Check of Philadelphia has been highlighted recently for his successful treatment of women with premature menopause. Doctors used to believe that no eggs remained in the ovary after premature menopause. Now they know that some dormant but potentially fertile eggs may be left in the ovaries of postmenopausal women. Dr. Check uses a high dose of estrogen to stimulate any egg follicles that are present. About 20 percent of the women who have the hormone treatments become pregnant, but only about 8 percent give birth. Unfortunately, a very high rate of miscarriage accompanies the treatment. The chance of a successful pregnancy after premature menopause is small, but new therapies like those used by Dr. Check at least provide an opportunity where none previously existed.

Instant Menopause

Hearts go out to the young women who experience an unexpected natural premature menopause. Too many of us forget, however, that the same loss is shared by thousands of young women who experience premature menopause when their ovaries are removed at the time of hysterectomy. At 32, Debbie and her husband Tom had one child and were planning to have at least one more. Debbie was, however, experiencing increasing pain from a condition known as endometriosis in which islands of cells that resemble those of the endometrium exist outside the uterus. Considerable pain can occur when these islands respond to the rise and fall of estrogen and progesterone and slough blood and debris into the abdominal cavity in synchrony with each menstrual period.

Debbie's condition did not respond satisfactorily to hormone and drug therapy. Her quality of life deteriorated due to recurring pain that caused her to miss work and other activities with increasing frequency. After long discussions with Tom and her physician, Debbie decided that a hysterectomy (surgical removal of the uterus) was imperative. Since endometriosis tissue surrounded her ovaries, they were also removed at the time of hysterectomy. Removal of her uterus put an end to her childbearing years; removal of her ovaries resulted in a *surgical menopause* or *instant menopause* that was also premature. Debbie had no climacteric, no perimenopause, no gradual period of adjustment to decreasing estrogen levels. Instant menopause can be accompanied by instant hot flashes, night sweats, vaginal dryness, irritability, absent-mindedness, or any of the other symptoms of natural menopause. Because the loss of estrogen is so abrupt, the symptoms are often even more intense. In the long term, surgical menopause can elevate the risk of osteoporosis and cardiovascular disease at a younger-than-normal age.

It is natural for women in their 20s, 30s, and 40s who are faced with hysterectomy to regret the loss of reproductive years that should have been theirs. These feelings were reflected in a recent article in *Patient Care* in which Drs. David Rudy and Irving Bush reported that some patients and their partners grieve the loss of the uterus as the symbol of motherhood. Even women who have completed their families sometimes feel pangs of loss at the finality of a hysterectomy. Regardless of age, women approaching a hysterectomy generally do so with some degree of anxiety and trepidation. These feelings of unrest diminish with time according to a British study in which 84 percent of the participating patients said that their general sense of well-being was much better 18 months after their hysterectomy than prior to the surgery.

Sex After Hysterectomy

The quality of sex after a hysterectomy is one issue that creates concern for most women and their partners when surgery is being considered. Couples naturally want to know if sex will be the same. Even though sex is a very important consideration, women frequently fail to ask the questions that are on their minds. What's more, the topic of sex after hysterectomy is not always addressed by the physician. Marvel Williamson discussed the difficult subject in a recent issue of the *Journal of Obstetrics, Gynecologic, and Neonatal Nursing*. She believes that the problem is considerable and that counseling concerning changes in sexual desire and function after hysterectomy is often ignored by physicians and nurses. The reason for the omission is not clear, but Williamson suggests some possibilities. Health-care professionals may find hysterectomy so routine that proper counseling is omitted as an oversight, or perhaps some physicians are uncomfortable discussing the subject of sexual adjustment after hysterectomy. Whatever the reason, Williamson believes that a physician's silence about sex can be detrimental to a patient's attitude about hysterectomy and subsequent sexual function. A woman may interpret a physician's lack of openness about sex after hysterectomy to mean that there is nothing to discuss, and jump to the conclusion that there is no sex life after hysterectomy. Nothing could be farther from the truth. During the 6 or so weeks following surgery, while tissues are healing, intercourse is not permitted. However, after the recovery period, sex can be as good as it was before hysterectomy. It is often better for women who have a hysterectomy to correct a painful condition caused by fibroids, endometriosis, or a prolapsed uterus.

There are, of course, physicians who go to an extreme when counseling patients about hysterectomy and sex. They maintain that hysterectomy does not affect sexuality at all. As a matter of fact, these doctors view any complaints or concerns about sex as psychological in origin. This attitude can also be harmful to a hysterectomy patient because it is not realistic. Sex after hysterectomy can be great, and while the uterus certainly isn't essential to sex, some women do notice subtle differences after it is removed. These changes are not imagined – they are real. During intercourse, the uterus changes shape and it also produces *prostaglandins* and *prostacyclins*. These substances play a role in maintaining vaginal tone and cause the vagina to change shape at orgasm. After the uterus is removed, not all women detect subtle differences in vaginal shape during intercourse. However, some women do. After hysterectomy, a woman and her partner may need to experiment with longer foreplay or different positions for intercourse, but hysterectomy should not affect the pleasure of an intimate relationship.

Other factors related to hysterectomy can affect a woman's sex life. When the ovaries are removed at the time of hysterectomy, a woman loses her main source of estrogen and testosterone. For some women, a drop in testosterone is accompanied by a sagging libido that results in a slump in her interest in sex. A team of Canadian researchers asked a group of women who had undergone hysterectomy and had their ovaries removed to stop all forms of hormone replacement therapy for four weeks. The researchers then surveyed the women and collected baseline data about the frequency of their sexual fantasies, sexual activity, and orgasm. The women were divided into three groups and given either estrogen replacement therapy, estrogen replacement therapy plus testosterone, or a placebo. After three weeks of treatment, the frequency of intercourse and orgasm had increased 4 to 6 times baseline levels in the women taking estrogen replacement therapy and testosterone. Women in the control group who received no hormone therapy showed a decline in sexual activity. Women in the estrogen replacement therapy group struck a happy medium. For them, the frequency of intercourse and orgasm rose to twice baseline levels. Most women find this a very acceptable level for their libido and for sexual activity.

How does estrogen bolster the libido? Remember that estradiol, estrone, and testosterone are very similar in molecular structure. Women who take estrogen replacement therapy and maintain a satisfactory sex drive probably have no problem converting some of the estrogen to testosterone. A few women find, however, that estrogen replacement therapy alone will not compensate for the loss of testosterone. Scientists are not sure why, but believe these women may lack the enzyme necessary to convert estrone to *dihydrotestosterone* (a form of testosterone). Women with this problem may realize a significant boost in their libido if a small amount of testosterone is added to their estrogen replacement therapy regimen.

Taking testosterone can have its drawbacks. Some women who use testosterone-containing preparations experience side effects that include liver problems, acne, edema, vaginal keratosis (thickening), changes in the texture and amount of body hair, and cigarette smokers may also suffer polycythemia (increased red blood cells). The side effects of testosterone are so unpleasant for some women that they opt to stop the therapy and contend with a diminished libido. The vast majority of women who have their ovaries removed at the time of hysterectomy begin estrogen replacement therapy to prevent transient symptoms like hot flashes and nausea and to control the long-term risks of osteoporosis and cardiovascular disease. This treatment is essential unless precluded by other health considerations like a history of breast cancer. The addition of testosterone to the therapy is a matter for each woman to consider with her partner and physician. Many women don't require testosterone, but those with a flagging libido may wish to at least give it a try.

Hysterectomy—Menopause to Follow

Sparing the ovaries at the time of hysterectomy leaves a premenopausal woman with her estrogen- and testosterone-producing systems intact. Physicians used to believe that the ovaries would continue to function normally and that menopause would then occur "on schedule" later in the woman's life. However, recent studies show that this is not the case. Probably 25 to 50 percent of the women who undergo hysterectomy with one or both ovaries spared have premature ovarian failure. Doctors are not sure why the ovaries shut down early. They speculate that the blood supply to the ovaries is disturbed during surgery and that this somehow shortens the active lifetime of these organs. Whatever the cause, early ovarian failure can be a reality. A 1987 study published in *Fertility and Sterility* compared the time of ovarian failure in women who had undergone hysterectomy with ovary preservation to age-matched women who had undergone natural menopause. The researchers used two main criteria to establish ovarian failure: persistent hot flashes intense enough to interfere with sleep and vaginal dryness severe enough to affect intercourse. The average age of ovarian failure was 45.4 years for women in the hysterectomy group and 49.4 years for women in the natural menopause group. The reason for early ovarian failure following hysterectomy remains under investigation.

Many physicians have been unaware of or slow to accept the reality of premature ovarian failure following hysterectomy. Sometimes several years elapse between hysterectomy and the onset of menopause and a woman "forgets" that menopause is still ahead. After hysterectomy, there are no menstrual periods, so irregular periods do not forewarn a woman as menopause approaches. Other early warning signs are often discounted or attributed to some other cause because a woman thinks she is "too young" for menopause. That's what happened to Donna. At age 33, she had a hysterectomy and one ovary was removed. The remaining ovary produced enough estrogen to ward off menopause for several years. Healthwise, her life was uneventful until age 45, when Donna went to her physician with a list of complaints. She had been irritable, depressed, fatigued, and hot all over for the previous 2 or 3 months. Donna was very fortunate. Her physician quickly recognized the symptoms of early ovarian failure even though Donna was younger than average for menopause. The ovarian failure was confirmed by an elevated FSH level. Subsequent estrogen replacement therapy brought Donna rapid relief from the symptoms of menopause. Unfortunately, Donna was typical of many women. After a few months of feeling like a new woman, she quit taking the prescribed estrogen. It was not long before the disturbing menopausal symptoms returned. Donna discussed her situation with her physician and realized that to be effective, estrogen replacement therapy usually needs to be a long-term therapy. Symptoms generally return if hormone therapy is discontinued as soon as a woman "feels better." As mentioned previously and discussed in detail in Chapter 8, the appropriate length of estrogen replacement therapy is still a matter of debate among physicians.

Hysterectomy — How Many and Why

More hysterectomies are performed in the United States than any other type of major surgery with the exception of cesarean section. Information from the National Center for Health Statistics indicates that more than one-third of American women will have a hysterectomy by age 60. Furthermore, according to data in the *Statistical Bulletin* (1989), young women aged 35 to 44 accounted for almost 40 percent of hysterectomies performed from 1985 through 1987. About 25 percent of the 650,000 hysterectomies performed in the United States each year are *nonelective surgeries* that are necessary to protect a woman's health. Nonelective hysterectomy can be required to stop severe hemorrhage, eliminate serious infection, or to correct certain other serious disorders that do not respond to other types of treatment. The majority of the nonelective hysterectomies or about 10 to 15 percent of all hysterectomies are prompted by precancerous cells or cancer cells in one of the reproductive organs. This is a modest proportion of the total number of the hysterectomies performed each year. Most women faced with a diagnosis of cancer in a reproductive organ are counseled to have a hysterectomy soon after diagnosis. However, there are a few exceptions. In some cases, it is prudent to first use other forms of treatment such as radiation therapy. For others, surgery is not advised because the cancer is extensive and has spread to other parts of the body, leaving no reasonable expectation that it can be removed.

Approximately 75 percent of the hysterectomies performed each year are not essential to save a woman's life. Instead, they are *elective surgeries* intended to relieve or eliminate symptoms of a number of reproductive organ diseases. The National Center for Health Statistics reports that more than two-thirds of all hysterectomies done in the United States are for fibroids, endometriosis, or uterine prolapse – generally not life-threatening conditions. These surgeries are primarily performed to reduce pain and improve the quality of a woman's life. In these situations, hysterectomy is a reasonable and appropriate choice.

There are physicians and health advocates who believe that some elective hysterectomies are unnecessary surgeries for conditions that could be satisfactorily treated by other methods. They point to lower rates of hysterectomy that are common throughout Europe and question the necessity of the large numbers of hysterectomies performed in this country. In the United States, 21 percent of women have had a hysterectomy by age 44. In contrast, a study carried out in six European countries found that only 4 percent had a hysterectomy by age 44.

Those who believe hysterectomy rates are excessive also direct attention to large differences in the number of surgeries performed in different geographic regions of the United States. Women living in the south and central states are 2 to 3 times more likely to have a hysterectomy than women living in the northeastern or west coast states. At present, there does not appear to be a satisfactory explanation for regional differences in the number of hysterectomies or for the high rates of surgery in the United States as compared to other countries.

Faced with a hysterectomy with or without removal of the ovaries, whether a nonelective, life-saving surgery or an elective procedure, a woman should know her options and consider them carefully. It is important to have a clear understanding of (1) why the hysterectomy is necessary or recommended, (2) what organs will be removed during the surgery, (3) whether alternative surgeries or treatments are available, (4) the risk of the surgery, (5) the impact of the surgery on future health and well-being, (6) the physical and emotional feelings that may precede or follow the surgery, (7) how estrogen levels will be changed, and (8) what sexual adjustments a woman and her partner may need to explore after surgery. Dr. Lisa McAdams, family practitioner in Nacogdoches, Texas, says it is not uncommon to take the medical history of a new patient who has had a previous hysterectomy but does not know why the surgery was performed or which organs were removed. A hysterectomy is a serious operation that usually involves a stay of about 6 days in the hospital and a recovery period of 6 or more weeks. A woman should know why she is undergoing such a serious procedure and what organs are to be removed. She should be informed even in the case of nonelective surgery where choices may be limited. It is her responsibility to be a participant in decisions concerning her health care.

Hysterectomy and Related Surgeries

Surgery to correct a problem concerning the female reproductive system was first performed by Ephraim McDowell in Danville, Kentucky, in 1809. McDowell removed a 22-pound ovarian cyst from a patient whose rather rapid recovery somewhat surprised him. But it is Charles Clay, a British surgeon, who is considered the real "father of ovariotomy" (removal of ovaries), even though his first surgery to remove an ovarian cyst was not performed until 1842. In the years that followed, however, Clay became so adept at the procedure he computed his surgeries by weight rather than number. The removal of 2000 pounds of ovarian tumors each month was apparently not unusual. Gynecologic surgeries are no longer reckoned in pounds of material removed and have evolved to include the removal or repair of the reproductive organs.

A procedure termed a *myomectomy* is less extensive than any of the hysterectomy procedures. It is sometimes selected to remove fibroid tumors or other benign growths from the uterus. It is more conservative than a hysterectomy since only the diseased portion of the uterus is removed. The remaining uterine tissue is reformed into a smaller but functional uterus that provides a woman with the option of having additional children. Some surgeons now perform this procedure through the vaginal opening, which greatly reduces the length of the hospital stay, recovery time, and expense.

There are four types of hysterectomy surgeries and all involve removal of the uterus. Only the fundus or top portion of the uterus is removed when a *subtotal hysterectomy* is performed. The cervix, which is the lower portion of the uterus, the Fallopian tubes, and the ovaries are left intact and the potential benefits of these organs are retained. Today, however, a subtotal hysterectomy is rarely if ever performed. Instead, a surgeon usually performs a *total hysterectomy* in which the entire uterus including the cervix is removed, but the Fallopian tubes and ovaries are left in place. Again, the potential benefit of continued production of estrogen from the ovaries is retained.

Removal of the uterus, cervix, both Fallopian tubes, and both ovaries is termed a *total hysterectomy with bilateral salpingo-oophorectomy* (bilateral = both sides, salpingo = Fallopian tube, oophor = ovary, ectomy = surgical removal) or more simply a *hysterectomy with oophorectomy*. When only one ovary is removed, the surgery is termed a hysterectomy with *unilateral salpingo-oophorectomy*. In either case, the vagina is retained but the woman's ability to have children is lost. Total hysterectomy with or without removal of one or both ovaries is the most common.

The number of women who have both ovaries removed at the time of hysterectomy is rising but occurs most frequently in females over 45. In the 20-year span between 1965 and 1985, the number of women aged 45 to 69 who had a hysterectomy with oophorectomy jumped from 35 percent to 66 percent. This reflects the trend among physicians to encourage women (not exclusively but especially those 45 and older) to have their ovaries removed at the time of hysterectomy. This is a prophylactic measure aimed at preventing future ovarian cancer. Ovarian cancer is a treacherous disease that basically has no warning signs and for which no reliable screening test exists. Removal of undiseased ovaries to ensure against the possibility of future ovarian cancer may be a very reasonable option, especially if a woman has completed her family and she is in a high-risk category for ovarian cancer. Some physicians argue that the threat of cancer of the ovaries is very small for most women and that they are better off keeping their ovaries and receiving the benefit of extra years of natural estrogen. The issue remains controversial and should be carefully considered with a physician.

There are cases, usually when cancer of the reproductive organs is quite extensive, when a *radical hysterectomy* is required in an attempt to lower the risk of subsequent cancer. This procedure includes a total hysterectomy with oophorectomy plus removal of considerable portions of the vagina. A radical hysterectomy is generally mandated by the type or extent of the cancer and leaves little if any room for options. A second opinion should always be sought when approaching any surgery.

Abdominal or Vaginal Surgery

When surgery to correct reproductive organ disease is necessary, there may be a choice concerning how the surgery is performed. An *abdominal hysterectomy* has been the long-time standard procedure. An abdominal incision is made, diseased organs are removed, and the incision is closed. Recovery time is often lengthy. Recently, surgeons have perfected a *vaginal hysterectomy* that does not require an abdominal incision and therefore reduces recovery time. In this procedure, some or all of the reproductive organs can be removed through the vaginal opening.

A *laparoscopic hysterectomy* is another procedure that reduces recovery time. In a laparoscopic procedure, a very small incision is made in the abdomen, usually at the navel, and a small tube is inserted through the incision. Gas is passed through the tube to inflate the abdomen and separate the organs. A thin fiber optic system is inserted to view the internal organs including the ovaries and the outside of the uterus and cervix. This procedure can be slow and tedious, since any material that is removed must be minced small enough to pass out through the laparoscopic tube. For this reason, laparoscopic hysterectomy is often limited to procedures that require removal of small amounts of material. As an alternative, laparoscopy is now sometimes combined with laser vaporization of small bits of material or with electrocauterization of material. These techniques can be very useful in the treatment of fibroids and endometriosis. The procedures are relatively new, and only a limited number of surgeons have developed the expertise to use them.

Quite recently, some surgeons have merged the laparoscopy and vaginal hysterectomy techniques with some truly remarkable results. The combined technique permits a surgeon to remove large fibroid tumors or extensive endometriosis tissue. Previously, these conditions required abdominal surgery in order to clearly see that all diseased tissue was removed. Vaginal surgery is now a very viable procedure for correction of these as well as many other disorders. The choice of hysterectomy or other treatment depends primarily on the type and extent of the reproductive disorder and on the expertise and experience of the surgeon. Hysterectomy may be the option of choice for cancer of the ovaries, Fallopian tubes, endometrium, or cervix. Hysterectomy may also be desirable to treat fibroid tumors, endometriosis, or a prolapsed uterus. Each of these conditions is considered below.

Ovarian Cancer

Approximately 20,000 women are diagnosed with ovarian cancer in the United States each year, and almost 12,800 die from the disease. It is most commonly detected in women aged 60 to 64 (some sources extend this age range to include women aged 55 to 74), but is not restricted to the postmenopausal age group. Diagnosis and treatment are complicated issues, because ovarian cancer is not a single disease. There are actually about 50 different types of ovarian cancer distinguished in part by the particular type of ovarian cell that is involved. Approximately 90 percent of all of the ovarian cancers involve the outer covering of the ovary and are classified as *epithelial ovarian cancer*. However, this category of cancer can be further subdivided into a number of different tumor types, making disease classification and treatment very complex.

A woman in the general U.S. population has a 1.7 percent chance of developing ovarian cancer, although rates among black women are universally low. Risk factors that contribute to the likelihood that a woman will suffer ovarian cancer include a history of menstrual problems, having no children or only one child, a high-fat diet, previous breast cancer, and obesity. A recent analysis of several studies comparing women with ovarian cancer to those without the disease suggests that certain fertility drugs may also pose the threat of an increased risk. The data, which recently appeared in the *American Journal of Epidemiology*, indicated an increased risk of ovarian cancer for women who had never been pregnant, had been diagnosed as infertile, and had been treated with the fertility drugs *Clomid* (*clomiphene*) or *Perganol* (*menotropins*). There appeared to be no increased risk of ovarian cancer for women who had been pregnant prior to taking the fertility drugs. The FDA urges caution in interpreting the results because the number of women included in the analysis was small (34 women with ovarian cancer and 23 women without), background information about the women and drugs was scant, and other similar studies have not linked the use of fertility drugs to ovarian cancer. Furthermore, 12.5 million courses of the drugs have been prescribed in the United States since the drugs were marketed in the late 1960s and early 1970s. In that time, only six cases of fertility-drug-related ovarian cancer have been reported to the FDA.

There is mounting evidence, however, that hormones may influence the development of ovarian cancer. Women who have had multiple pregnancies or taken birth control pills are at *reduced risk* for ovarian cancer. The Cancer and Steroid Hormone Study by the Centers for Disease Control and The National Institute of Child Health and Human Services reported that the use of oral contraceptives for even a few months reduced the risk of ovarian cancer by 40 percent in women aged 20 to 54 years. The study also found that the risk continued to decrease the longer a woman remained on birth control pills. Because of these data, a lowered incidence of ovarian cancer is now listed among the noncontraceptive health benefits on oral contraceptive labels.

Familial or *inherited ovarian cancer* is estimated to account for only about 5 to 10 percent of the total number of cases. It is this inherited form of ovarian cancer that is often diagnosed in younger women. As noted above, most women have a 1.7 percent chance of developing ovarian cancer during their lifetime. A woman's risk increases if she has a mother or sister who has ovarian cancer and jumps to approximately 40 percent if two or more immediate family members are diagnosed with the disease. The Familial Ovarian Cancer Registry at Roswell Park Cancer Institute in Buffalo, New York, listed 2144 cases of ovarian cancer in 899 families as of April 1992. The organization urges women who have two or more close family members (mother, sister, daughter, grandmother, aunt) with ovarian cancer to seek genetic counseling beginning in their early 20s and to have physical checkups every six months beginning in their early 30s. These should include pelvic and abdominal examinations, tests for the level of CA 125 (a substance commonly elevated in women with some forms of advanced ovarian cancer), and pelvic or transvaginal ultrasound examinations. The Registry also recommends that women in this group who have completed their families undergo prophylactic removal of their ovaries by age 35.

The genes that impact on ovarian cancer are not well understood, but headway is being made in determining the role that some genes play in the disease's progress. A recent study led by Dr. Dennis Slamon found that 25 percent of women with ovarian cancer had extra copies of a special gene called *HER-2/neu*. These women were much less responsive to standard treatments and had shorter survival times.

There are rarely early warning signs that signal the presence of ovarian cancer, although abdominal pain or abnormal uterine bleeding may occur. When symptoms are present, they are frequently vague and difficult to distinguish from those of a number of other diseases. Furthermore, there are no reliable diagnostic tests for ovarian cancer so it is most often detected in advanced stages. Lack of reliable screening tests and ambiguous symptoms often result in prolonged periods of testing and analysis prior to diagnosis. Gilda Radner, one of the original Not-Ready-for-Prime-Time Players on the "Saturday Night Live" television show, had such an experience. She believed something was wrong long before she learned that she had ovarian cancer. In her book, *It's Always Something*, she recounts her frustration and anxiety during the 10 months that eventually resulted in a diagnosis of cancer of the ovaries.

The real key to decreasing the rates of ovarian cancer is early detection. Researchers searching for a reliable screening test to detect ovarian cancer in early stages have developed some promising techniques. *Transvaginal ultrasound* is a helpful diagnostic tool that employs an ultrasound probe placed in the vagina, within millimeters of the ovaries. Screening for *CA 125*, a substance found in elevated amounts in some patients with advanced ovarian cancer, may also prove effective. The National Cancer Institute is currently conducting a clinical trial of 74,000 women aged 60 to 74 to determine the value of transvaginal ultrasound and CA 125 for early detection of ovarian cancer. A 1993 article in the *New England Journal of Medicine* written by Dr. D. L. Healy and colleagues reported elevated levels of the hormone inhibin in most women with certain types of ovarian cancer. Inhibin levels may prove to be a valuable diagnostic tool for these particular tumors since they are not associated with high levels of CA 125.

Diagnosis often occurs after a tumor is detected as an enlarged ovary at the time of pelvic examination, but by then the cancer is in an advanced stage. Ovarian cancer grows rapidly, has easy access to other abdominal organs, and spreads quickly. Treatment usually consists of removing the uterus, Fallopian tubes, and ovaries if the cancer is not so extensive as to be inoperable. Both ovaries are normally removed even when only one shows signs of disease, because cancer in one ovary is usually followed by cancer in the other. Postsurgical radiation therapy or chemotherapy with *cyclophosphamide* (*Cytoxan*) in combination with a platinum-containing drug like *carboplatin* (*Paraplatin*) or *cisplatin* (*Platinol*) may also be required. Following surgery, chemotherapy, and/or radiation therapy, some physicians perform a *laparotomy* or "second-look surgery." The surgeon inserts a *laporascope*, a flexible, lighted tube, through a small incision in the abdomen and can see the internal organs and remove small pieces of tissue for biopsy. This procedure permits a better evaluation of the effectiveness of chemotherapy and radiation therapy.

Taxol, a new experimental drug derived from the bark of the Pacific yew tree, *Taxus brevifola*, is showing great promise in the treatment of advanced and recurrent ovarian cancer as well as breast cancer. In 1992, the National Cancer Institute authorized the use of taxol for ovarian cancer under a special program that permits earlier and wider access to experimental drugs by patients with life-threatening diseases for which no satisfactory treatment exists. The results of the taxol clinical trials, which are anticipated to include over 6000 patients, may provide sound scientific basis for widespread use of taxol as a weapon against ovarian cancer.

Cancer of the Fallopian Tubes

Cancer of the Fallopian tubes, the rarest of the reproductive organ cancers, generally involves the cells that line the Fallopian tubes. In about 15 percent of the cases, both Fallopian tubes are involved. Like ovarian cancer, it is difficult to detect, may be asymptomatic, and is often in advanced stages and has spread to other abdominal organs when diagnosed. Possible symptoms are pelvic or abdominal pain, abnormal vaginal bleeding, and vaginal discharge. Treatment is similar to that for ovarian cancer. If the disease has not spread and surgery is recommended, both ovaries and Fallopian tubes are removed as well as the uterus. Subsequent radiation therapy is also often required.

Uterine or Endometrial Cancer

Uterine cancer strikes 38,000 women in the United States each year. Although the primary age group ranges from 50 to 55 years, women of any age are susceptible. This is another cancer that can be hereditary, so risks are highest for women with a mother or a sister who has had uterine cancer. Additional risk factors are similar to those for ovarian cancer and include a history of menstrual problems, having no children or only one child, a high-fat diet, previous breast cancer, and obesity.

Uterine cancer frequently originates in the endometrium and is therefore often referred to as *endometrial cancer*. It grows slowly and generally remains confined to the endometrium and the inside of the uterus until advanced stages are reached. According to the American Cancer Society, efficient early detection methods and the slow growth of the cancer result in over 80 percent of uterine cancer cases being diagnosed while the disease is still limited to the uterus. Consequently, the cure rate is excellent (50 to 70 percent), and the annual death rate is low (3000 women).

Treatment of uterine cancer in an early stage before it has spread usually consists of surgery to remove the uterus, Fallopian tubes, and ovaries, and in some cases the cervix and pelvic lymph nodes. More advanced stages of the cancer may also require removal of part of the vagina and sometimes other nearby tissues.

The surgery is generally followed by radiation therapy, which may be a critical part of the cure for many women. A recent issue of *Geriatrics* summarized a retrospective study by Dr. Sameer Rafla, director of radiation oncology at Methodist Hospital in Brooklyn, New York. Dr. Rafla and colleagues found that women who received about 5 weeks of daily radiation postoperatively had a 5-year survival rate or "cure rate" of over 90 percent. This was true even when the cancer had spread to the cervix or penetrated through the endometrium. Patients with similar endometrial cancers who did not receive radiation therapy did poorly by comparison. They had a 5-year survival rate of 50 percent or less.

Cancer of the Cervix

Cervical cancer strikes women of all ages and is frequent in those 35 and younger. Risk factors for cervical cancer include early first intercourse, multiple sex partners, and infection with the human papillomavirus (HPV), which is sexually transmitted. Only 3 percent of HPV-positive women develop cervical cancer, but more and more evidence indicates that HPV infection is a significant risk factor for developing the disease. Smoking is another factor that may increase the risk of cervical cancer, perhaps by as much as 50 percent for some women.

Recent media stories have incorrectly given the alarming impression that the rates of cervical cancer are on the rise. Experts at the National Cancer Institute and the Centers for Disease Control and Prevention have been quick to point out that this is simply a case of confusing numbers. Baby boomers are swelling the ranks of young women, creating an increase in the number of cases of cervical cancer being reported. However, the actual rate of cervical cancer has been decreasing over the past years and is now fairly stable. About 13,000 women are diagnosed with cervical cancer each year. (Compare this to the 186,000 cases of breast cancer that are diagnosed annually.) More important, the death rate from cancer of the cervix has plummeted by 70 percent in the last 50 years and rests at a current level of 4400 women each year.

Much of the credit for this precipitous drop in deaths from cervical cancer goes to Dr. George Papanicolaou, who developed the painless, inexpensive way to detect early precancerous changes in cervical cell struc-ture that allows cervical cancer to be avoided. The procedure is called a *Pap smear* or *Pap test* after Dr. Papanicolaou. A physician usually uses a small brush called a *cytobrush* to collect cells from the "transformation zone." This is the line of demarcation between the tissue on the surface of the cervix and the tissue lining the cervical canal. A sample contains 50,000 to 300,000 cells that are literally smeared onto a glass slide that is sent to a specialized laboratory to be examined by certified technicians for the pres-ence of abnormal cells. Even though the test is fairly accurate, results that indicate abnormal changes when cancer is not present do occur with some regularity. Consequently, only a small number of cases that have abnormal cells actually result in a diagnosis of cervical cancer. There are a number of probable reasons for this: in 1989, terminology for the reporting system changed, possibly resulting in more minor cellular changes being classified as atypical; sometimes samples are inadequate for analysis; and sometimes "minor" changes disappear on re-examination. An abnormal Pap smear should not be alarming but should be followed up by a physician. Yet Martha Romans, director of the Jacobs Institute of Women's Health in Washington, D.C., finds that only about 60 percent of women with abnor-mal Pap smears return for a follow-up test.

There are a few general guidelines to keep in mind before getting a Pap test that can optimize results. It is suggested that Pap tests be performed 10 to 14 days after the first day of the last menstrual period although this is not mandatory. It is best not to douche for several days beforehand or use any vaginal medications, lubricants, or spermicides for at least 24 hours preceding the examination. The chemicals in these substances can alter cervical cells and make the tests difficult to interpret. Intercourse is okay if contraception does not require a vaginal spermicide.

There seems little doubt that the Pap test could save more lives through early detection of cervical cancer if only more women were aware of its benefits. At a recent conference marking the 50th anniversary of the Pap test, Michael Bower, vice president of Bruskin Goldring Research, pre-sented the results of a survey on women's knowledge, attitude, and behav-ior toward Pap testing. Of the women surveyed, 37 percent did not recall having an annual Pap test and 25 percent could not give a reason for having a Pap test. In addition, the survey uncovered many misconceptions about the Pap test. For example, 17 percent of the women could not name any specific cancer found by the test and 7 percent thought it detected breast cancer. Educational information concerning the importance of the Pap test as an early diagnostic tool is essential.

Abnormalities that are detected early can often be treated by removal of a small part of the cervix. In these cases, the woman retains her fertility and the ability to have children following surgery. Additional examinations, including Pap smears, are necessary to monitor the cervix and assure that all the diseased tissue has been removed. Advanced cases of cervical cancer require radiation therapy and/or hysterectomy. The treatment depends on the extent of the cancer and whether or not it has spread to other reproductive organs.

The American Cancer Society and the American College of Obstetricians and Gynecologists recommend that all women who are or have been sexually active have an annual Pap test and pelvic examination. Although it is controversial, some authorities believe that after three consecutive normal results, the test may be done less often if the woman and her doctor agree. Women at high risk should have an annual Pap test even when test results are consistently normal. According to a 1992 article in *Annals of Internal Medicine*, the incidence of cervical cancer remains higher among older women who are less likely to have gynecological examinations on a regular basis. It is estimated that cervical cancer deaths in older women could be reduced by 74 percent if women over 65 who have not had regular Pap smears in younger years were to get tested every three years. On the other hand, women aged 65 and older who have a history of negative Pap smears seem to be at very low risk. Some authorities recommend that these women discontinue Pap tests. Advice concerning the frequency of Pap tests can be confusing and should be discussed with a physician.

Fibroid Tumors of the Uterus

There are usually limited choices in the treatment of cancer of the reproductive organs. Other reproductive disorders, including fibroid tumors, endometriosis, and prolapsed uterus, can be serious but sometimes offer a greater degree of latitude in treatment.

It is estimated that approximately 20 percent of all women and 25 percent of women over the age of 35 have *fibroid tumors* or *uterine leiomyomas*. Fibroid tumors are most commonly diagnosed, however, in women in their 30s and 40s. These tumors apparently arise from the muscle tissue of the uterine wall and are benign or noncancerous over 99 percent of the time. They generally occur in clusters, with individual tumors ranging from pea-size to grapefruit-size or larger. The tumors themselves are harmless, but they can interfere with other structures and create serious problems that include enlarging the abdomen, abdominal discomfort or pain, abnormally long or heavy menstrual periods, scar tissue, and infertility. Large fibroids can also create pressure on the bladder, causing urinary frequency, or they may press on the rectum and result in constipation. In addition, large fibroids in the uterus can interfere with normal healing of the endometrium after menstruation and cause minimal to profuse, uncontrollable hemorrhage. In cases of severe hemorrhage or unbearable pain, immediate nonelective surgery may be required. This situation occurs, but is not common. Generally there is time to investigate options and make an informed choice between surgery and alternative therapies.

Since fibroid growth appears to be stimulated at least in part by estrogen, problematic tumors may shrink after menopause, when estrogen production declines. Prior to menopause, hormone treatments are available that can shrink the tumors and alleviate the distress if symptoms are moderate. *RU 486*, the controversial French morning-after pill, has been used for this purpose in a study by Dr. Ana Murphy, a gynecologist at the University of California at San Diego. She found that given orally, RU 486 acts by suppressing progesterone production and dramatically reduces the size of fibroids without serious side effects. After the RU 486 treatment, most of the patients in the group studied by Dr. Murphy had a myomectomy.

The combination of drug therapy to shrink fibroids followed by myomectomy also works with other drugs. *Lupron*, another new drug, shrinks fibroids by suppressing estrogen production. Lupron also causes side effects that can include hot flashes, vaginal dryness, and, over a long term of treatment, bone loss. Lupron is not a permanent cure for fibroids since they grow back to their former size when drug therapy is discontinued. However, like RU 486 Lupron can be useful for shrinking fibroids prior to surgical removal. Elective hysterectomy may be the most reasonable consideration if hormone treatments are ineffective, if fibroids return after myomectomy, or if fibroids are very large. Again, desire for future children and age until menopause are two of the many factors that should be carefully considered and discussed with a physician.

Endometriosis

It is estimated that approximately 15 percent of the female population or as many as 1 in 7 menstruating women has *endometriosis*. It is a condition in which islands of cells very much like the endometrial cells that line the uterus are found on the outer surfaces of the uterus, ovaries, Fallopian tubes, or less commonly on the rectum, bladder, or other organs within the abdominal cavity. The origin of the tissue is uncertain, but many researchers think that a process called *retrograde menstruation* is responsible. According to this conjecture, some of the normal menstrual fluid flows backwards, leaves the uterus through the Fallopian tubes, and enters the abdominal cavity. Other scientists suggest that the cells are "misplaced" in the abdominal cavity during fetal development. They speculate that these cells differentiate during puberty or early adulthood. Some unusual differences can be seen when the cells of the endometrial islands are compared to normal endometrial cells using the electron microscope. These differences leave the issue of the origin of the islands of endometrial cells unresolved.

Regardless of origin, the misplaced cells do respond to the same monthly changes in hormone levels that affect the endometrial lining of the uterus. These islands of cells grow and then shed on the same schedule as the endometrium, but the shed tissue and blood has no exit route from the abdominal cavity. The debris and blood that accumulate can be slight and go unnoticed or can be substantial and cause extreme pain. These renegade islands of cells can create additional problems. Like true endometrial cells, they have the ability to release prostaglandins that can cause spasms of the smooth muscles in the uterus and result in painful menstrual-like cramps. Prostaglandins can also stimulate contractions of the intestines and cause diarrhea and/or nausea.

Symptoms of endometriosis sometimes begin during puberty but more frequently are noticed later in the reproductive years after the islands of tissue have grown. Some women with the condition are unaware of it until the endometriosis is discovered during surgery for other reasons. Other women have mild discomfort, and a few suffer with extremely painful menstrual periods. The Endometriosis Association surveyed 3000 women and found the most common complaints by women with endometriosis were painful periods (96%), pelvic pain at other times of the month (83%), bowel problems during menstruation including cramping, diarrhea, constipation, or blood in stool (79%), heavy or irregular bleeding (65%), painful intercourse (60%), and dizziness, headaches, or nausea during menstruation (59%). The problems sometimes subside at menopause when hormone levels naturally decrease, but can continue in women taking hormone replacement therapy.

Treatment usually depends on the degree of discomfort. Women with minimal discomfort may need no treatment or may get relief from an analgesic or anti-inflammatory agent like *ibuprofen*. More severe symptoms often respond to drugs or hormone preparations that suppress the cyclic changes in the endometrial islands of cells. Many options are now available, including oral contraceptives, progestins, and compounds that mimic the action of gonadotropin-releasing hormone. *Danocrine* (*danazol*) is a synthetic hormone that is used to shrink the endometrial islands of cells. A recent study at Harvard Medical School in Boston reported that Danocrine improved symptoms in 89 percent of the patients studied and reduced the size or number of the endometrial islands in 94 percent. However, endometriosis recurred within five years in about one-third of the patients. The drug has side effects that include weight gain, decreased breast size, and a deepened voice. *Synarel* (*nafarelin acetate*), a drug dispensed as a nasal spray, also relieves symptoms and/or shrinks endometriosis islands. Again, endometriosis and its symptoms recur in many women when treatment is stopped. The side effects of Synarel include those typical of menopause— hot flashes, vaginal dryness, and lighter or absent periods. *Lupron Depot* (*leuprolide acetate*) has been approved for treatment of endometriosis as well as fibroids. It is given in monthly injections for six months and has side effects similar to those of Synarel. Like Danocrine and Synarel, the curative effects often reverse after treatment is stopped.

Drug intervention does not always provide adequate therapy. Women whose symptoms persist at a level that infringes on their quality of life may choose to have surgery to remove the islands of endometrial cells. If the endometrial islands are limited in number and not too extensive in size, laparoscopy is sometimes used to see the implants that can be removed by excision, laser vaporization, or electrocautery. In some cases, laparoscopy allows the surgeon to preserve the reproductive organs. This is an important consideration to young women who wish to have more children. Laparoscopy has the additional benefits of a minimal stay in the hospital and a brief recovery period at home.

Sometimes, however, the extent of the endometrial tissue is so great that hysterectomy is the only viable option to alleviate pain and psychological stress. This is a significant decision that should be carefully considered, keeping in mind the desire for additional children and age until menopause. However, elective hysterectomy may be a very appropriate choice to correct a severe case of endometriosis.

Prolapsed Uterus

Prolapsed uterus is another condition that is sometimes corrected by hysterectomy. It is common in women who have had several children and women who have passed menopause. Prolapse occurs when the muscles that normally hold the uterus in position above the cervix and between the bladder and rectum become weakened. The compromised muscles allow the uterus to sag into the cervix and impinge on the bladder. A prolapsed uterus can contribute to urinary incontinence because the condition weakens the bladder and decreases its capacity. Early detection and therapy are important since prolapse becomes more serious if left unattended.

Early stages of prolapsed uterus can sometimes be corrected by exercises to strengthen the muscles that support the uterus. This option can be discussed with a gynecologist, although some authorities maintain that the exercises are most effective when taught by an expert in biofeedback. They use special instrumentation to ensure that the correct muscles are working and to assess progress. In some cases, surgery to "resuspend" the uterus may be an option that can bring relief from the symptoms of prolapse. However, in severe cases, elective hysterectomy may be the best solution to a difficult problem. Again, this is a situation that requires thoughtful consideration and consultation with a physician.

6

The
Silent
Epidemic

Fragile Bones

It is difficult to ignore menopause symptoms like hot flashes and vaginal dryness, but *osteoporosis*, one of the more serious consequences of menopause, often proceeds unnoticed for years. Unfortunately, what you don't feel can hurt you. Osteoporosis accelerates the gradual rate of bone loss that is normal as one ages. This silent disease eats away at bones, leaving them porous, brittle, and very fragile. The bone that is left is normal, but sometimes there is not enough of it to maintain the integrity of the skeleton and support the body's weight.

Dwindling estrogen supplies contribute to bone deterioration, which is greatest in the 5 to 10 years that follow menopause. Bone is lost at a rate of about 2 percent per year during the first 5 years after menopause. Then the pace gradually slows and plateaus at a rate of 1 percent per year. A loss of 1 or 2 percent of bone mass each year may seem small, but by age 60 many women have lost 15 to 20 percent of their bone mass. Osteoporosis can cause the erosion of bone to be so great that the stress of rising from a chair can break a hip or bending over to pick up the morning newspaper can fracture a vertebra.

Osteoporosis officially holds the unenviable status of *the most common chronic-health condition among women over 45 years of age* and is estimated to affect as many as 50 percent of the women in this age group. The weakened bones that result from osteoporosis clearly pose a major health threat to the 20 million postmenopausal women who suffer 1.3 million bone fractures annually. Approximately 50,000 of these women die each year, usually from complications following hip fractures. Many others who suffer fractures experience a loss of independence and a dramatically decreased quality of life.

Because osteoporosis proceeds with no early warning signs, it is important that women confront the challenge of this menopause-related threat by being informed. Basic knowledge of bone structure and the process that continually replaces bone allows one to understand how osteoporosis weakens the skeleton, why fractures of the wrist, spine, and hip become increasingly common after menopause, and how to slow the pace of bone loss.

Bare Bone Facts

Bone is living tissue that from childhood on is constantly being renewed and repaired by a process called *bone remodeling*. The bone remodeling process also releases calcium, a major component of bone, when it is needed for other body functions like nerve transmission, muscle contraction, and blood clotting. The mechanism that initiates and terminates the release of calcium from bone is controlled by two hormones, *parathyroid hormone* and *calcitonin*.

Body sensors monitor the amount of calcium in the bloodstream and trigger the release of parathyroid hormone when calcium levels are low. The hormone activates large cells called *osteoclasts* that destroy bone tissue and release entrapped calcium. As the body's needs for calcium are met, the osteoclasts carve a small cavity in the bone called a *bone remodeling unit*. When circulating levels of calcium become excessive, body sensors trigger the thyroid gland to release the hormone calcitonin, which stops further removal of calcium from the bone. Calcium-containing bone cells called *osteoblasts* arise from the bone marrow and build new bone to replace the bone removed by the osteoclasts. Before age 35, the bone remodeling process works efficiently and bone is added faster than it is removed. In a woman's early years, the whole process of bone removal and replacement in one bone remodeling unit normally takes about four months. Bone remodeling units are quite small, but, because they are numerous, scientists estimate that between 10 and 30 percent of a person's entire skeleton is renewed each year in this piecemeal fashion.

Bone reaches maximum density at about age 35. After that, the bone remodeling process slowly loses efficiency and bone is removed faster than it is replaced. This accounts for the gradual loss of a small amount of total bone mass that is considered normal as a person ages. However, osteoporosis slows the bone remodeling process tremendously, causing the erosion and rebuilding of one bone remodeling unit to require up to 2 years or 6 times longer than usual. Bone loss is favored over bone rebuilding by such a large margin that bones become very fragile and often break under minor stresses.

The Estrogen Connection

Estrogen replacement therapy counteracts the devastation of osteoporosis by decreasing the rate of bone loss. The precise role that estrogen plays in slowing osteoporosis is not known, but researchers have suggested that estrogen may decrease bone turnover by inhibiting the action or number of osteoclasts that form bone remodeling units. Estrogen therapy first slows resorption or loss of bone and allows ongoing remodeling cycles to be completed. In addition, fewer new cycles are started, so bone loss stops or significantly slows down. Very recently, researchers have identified estrogen receptors in the nuclei of the bone-building osteoblasts. It seems likely that estrogen may play a direct regulatory function in the activities of these cells, but such a role has not yet been established.

In 1981, a group of scientists at the University of Copenhagen were among the first to clearly show that estrogen replacement therapy protects bone mass and apparently promotes new bone growth. The 114 women in the study were 6 months to 3 years past menopause. The volunteers were randomly divided into two groups. One group received a combination therapy of estrogen and progestin and gained an average of 3.7 percent in bone mass in their forearm. A second group of women received a placebo and lost an average of 5.7 percent of their forearm bone mass. After 18 months, half of the women receiving hormone therapy and gaining bone mass were switched to a placebo. These women began to lose bone mass while those who kept receiving hormone therapy continued to maintain their bone mass. The converse was also true. Half of the women who had been receiving a placebo for 18 months and losing bone were switched to hormone therapy and began to gain bone mass. The women who remained on a placebo throughout the 3-year experiment never experienced an increase in bone mass. The investigators concluded that estrogen can halt the process of bone loss and even promote bone formation in postmenopausal women.

Many recent studies support the data from this early investigation and confirm that estrogen plays a significant role in slowing the rate of bone loss due to osteoporosis. For example, in a report in a 1992 issue of *Obstetrics and Gynecology*, a group of Danish physicians described a 2-year study in which they compared changes in bone density in 62 healthy women who were 6 months to 3 years past menopause. The women were divided into groups. One group received a combination of estrogen and progestin; the other group received a placebo. The women given hormones lost no bone density in the wrist bones and gained 3 to 4 percent in bone density in the spine. The women receiving the placebo lost 5 to 6 percent of their wrist bone density and 2 percent of their bone density in the spine. Clearly, 2 or 3 years of estrogen therapy enhances bone density in postmenopausal women.

Other research shows that long-term estrogen therapy provides benefits that last several years past menopause by maintaining bone density and reducing the likelihood of fractures. Dr. David Felson, of the Boston University Arthritis Center, and colleagues have reported the protective effects in women who took estrogen for seven or more years. In women less than 75 years old who had taken estrogen for 7 or more years, the average bone density was 11.2 percent greater than that of women who had never taken estrogen. Among women who were 75 years of age or older, estrogen users (7 or more years) had an average bone density that was 3.2 percent higher than that of women who had never taken estrogen. Women who took estrogen for less than 7 years did not realize these long-term benefits in increased bone density that translate into decreased risk of fracture. Data from another study emphasized the positive benefit of estrogen to bone strength in postmenopausal women. Women 65 to 74 who were past estrogen users had a 63 percent reduction in the risk of hip fracture while women older than 75 had an 18 percent reduced risk when compared to women who had never taken estrogen. Investigators have found that when estrogen replacement therapy is stopped, even after several years, rapid loss of bone mass resumes and the risk of fracture increases accordingly. These data have led some experts to believe that continued use of estrogen for life is warranted to protect against the risk of fractures due to osteoporosis. Long-term protection against cardiovascular disease may be an added benefit.

Calcium

Estrogen not only protects against loss of bone density, it also has a significant effect on the amount of calcium the body has available to build bones. Estrogen therapy significantly increases the uptake of calcium from the gastrointestinal tract of estrogen-deficient women and decreases the loss of calcium by excretion. This is another important role for estrogen since each day the body must take in more calcium than it uses or loses in urine, feces, or sweat to stay in *positive calcium balance*. A *negative calcium* balance results when more calcium is used or lost than is supplied in the diet. In this situation, bone tissue must be broken down to meet demands for other body functions. A negative calcium balance as small as 30 mg/day (less than the amount in 1 ounce of milk) can lead to the loss of one-third of a person's bone mass over a 30-year period. A larger calcium deficit would presumably hasten bone loss.

Calcium is so vital to bone formation that, for a while, it was thought that calcium alone might protect against significant bone loss. A number of studies like the one recently reported in *Obstetrics and Gynecology* by Drs. Robert Lindsay and Jack Tohme of Columbia University in New York show that this is not the case. A group of 50 women who had osteoporosis and were about 14 years past menopause participated in a study to evaluate the effects of calcium and estrogen on bone density. Half of the women received daily 1500-mg calcium supplements. The other half received the calcium supplement plus estrogen replacement therapy. After 2 years, the women who received only a calcium supplement had lost bone density in the vertebrae and in the hip while the estrogen-plus-calcium group gained bone density at both sites. The study clearly demonstrated that calcium alone cannot effectively protect against bone loss.

A Move in the Right Direction

Exercise is one of the best all-around promoters of general health and is essential for maintaining bone strength. Inactivity has just the opposite effect and invites bone loss. One team of researchers demonstrated the

importance of exercise on bone density by convincing a group of participants with normal bone density to rest in bed, simulating patients temporarily immobilized for fracture or illness. The volunteers stayed in bed for
11 to 61 days. At the end of the bed-rest trial, the participants had all lost
bone from their vertebrae. The longer they rested, the more bone they
lost. This type of bone loss is initially rather rapid, then slows down.
Unlike losses from osteoporosis, these deficits in bone density usually
recover once activity is resumed.

While inactivity promotes bone loss, exercise, particularly weight-
bearing activity, enhances bone strength and reduces bone loss in women
with osteoporosis. Studies of several age groups indicate that physically
active people have denser bones than less active people in the same age
group. Some of the best exercises to fight osteoporosis are also some of the
simplest. Walking, jogging, hiking, running, biking, rowing, jumping rope,
or climbing stairs are excellent weight-bearing exercises that promote strong
bones, increase muscle tone, and benefit the cardiovascular and respiratory
systems. The amount of exercise necessary to foster bone formation and
maintain healthy bones is not known. Exercising every day is excellent for
those who have the time and inclination. Exercising 3 to 4 times a week
for 10 to 15 minutes, slowly working up to 20 or 30 minutes, is a realistic
goal that provides proven benefit.

Unfortunately, women who already have severe osteoporosis or arthritis
may find it uncomfortable to do even the simplest weight-bearing exercises.
Swimming, although not a weight-bearing exercise, is a good alternative
activity that provides some resistance without placing undue stress on
already weakened bones. It also benefits the cardiovascular and respiratory
systems, promotes muscle tone, and increases muscle strength.

Exercise is important to bone health, but a recent report indicates that
by itself, it is not sufficient to maintain bone density in postmenopausal
women. A group of 120 postmenopausal women (mean age, 54) with low
bone density in their forearms were divided into three experimental groups.
One group exercised, another exercised and took a calcium supplement,
and the third group exercised and received estrogen replacement therapy
(with progestin as necessary). The three groups and a control group of 42
women with normal forearm bone density were followed for two years.
The women in the exercise and control groups lost about the same amount
of bone. Women in the exercise plus calcium group also lost bone but not
quite as much. The women in the exercise plus estrogen group had a

significant increase in bone density in their forearms. Strong evidence indicates that a combination of estrogen replacement therapy, adequate calcium, and moderate weight-bearing exercise is the most successful regimen for maintaining bone density after menopause.

Broken Bones

Not all bones are created equally, so postmenopausal women do not usually break an arm or a leg. The shafts of these long bones are protected with a thick outer layer of *compact bone* that is quite dense and contains few spaces. This natural density allows compact bone to withstand rapid weakening by osteoporosis and these bones remain relatively "fracture-resistant." Wrist, spine, hip, and rib bones are composed primarily of *spongy bone tissue*. These bones account for the greatest number of osteoporosis-related fractures. Spongy bone is made of a crisscrossed lattice work of bony girders that surround rather large spaces filled with blood-cell-producing bone marrow. Spongy bone is quite strong in its prime, but the supportive bony girders are quickly eroded and weakened by osteoporosis. Eventually a woman may lose about half of her spongy bone. It is not surprising that fractures of the wrist, spine, hip, and rib bones increase with age.

Wrist or *Colle's fractures* are the most common type of fracture among white women under 75 years of age. Many of these occur when a woman puts out her hand to break a fall. Wrist fractures can be painful, but they generally have few long-term consequences. On the other hand, fractures of the spine and hip are frequently associated with continuing problems.

The National Arthritis Workgroup estimates that 24 to 25 million women aged 45 years and older have osteoporosis of the spine. As a consequence, one in three women over 50 will suffer a vertebral fracture. Normally, each vertebra is shaped like a tiny rectangular box. An initial compression fracture usually crushes a vertebra on one side, forming it into a wedge with the crushed side toward the front of the body. The bulk of the body's weight is situated in front of the spine, which puts extreme stress on this side of the vertebrae. It also pulls on already fractured vertebrae and deforms the entire spine into a curve. Additional stress may cause a wedge-shaped vertebra to fracture again and collapse on itself so that it resembles a flattened box. It is estimated that each vertebral compression fracture reduces a person's height by about ½ cm or ¼ inch. Women with several vertebral compression fractures lose as much as 2 to 8 inches in height and are characterized by a dowager's hump, a condition medically termed *kyphosis*. This classic symptom of osteoporosis is only apparent in the end stages of the disease and is generally associated with chronic pain.

However, the most serious consequences of osteoporosis are the more than 300,000 hip fractures that occur every year. There are several types of fractures of the bones of the hip that get lumped into one catch-all category termed hip fracture. The most common types occur in the upper end of the femur, which is the large bone in the thigh. Hip fractures sometimes occur from a physical stress as minimal as rising from a chair. The fracture usually causes a fall that gets the blame for the broken hip. The threat of this type of fracture can be reduced if the stress on hip joints is minimized by using both hands to push down on the chair seat or arms when standing. A 1994 study headed by Dr. Susan Greenspan who is associated with Beth Israel Hospital and Harvard University reports that falls to the side significantly increased the risk of hip fracture in the group studied. She stresses the importance of eliminating environmental hazards such as throw rugs, cords, poorly lit stairways, and high-heeled shoes. Hip padding, appropriate diet, and leg exercises are also recommended measures to guard against hip fracture.

Some women do not realize they have broken a hip until several hours after a fall. Katherine's story is a good example. At age 69 (well below the median age for hip fracture), Katherine felt fine, was active, and had no dowager's hump or other visible symptoms of osteoporosis. She was returning to her car after a typical shopping trip when she fell and injured her right hip. The fall seemed minor, so Katherine continued home. The following day, her discomfort was so great that she went to see her doctor. X rays confirmed that Katherine's minor fall had resulted in a broken hip. Katherine is just one of many victims of the silent epidemic who show no outward symptoms of bone loss until a bone breaks from some minor stress.

After menopause, the rate of hip fracture doubles with each 10-year increase in age. Different investigators place the median age of hip fracture either late in the eighth decade or in the ninth decade of life. This is just an average, however, and many women like Katherine suffer a hip fracture long before they are 80 years old. Hip fractures often result in complications related to surgery or from being confined to bed. Each year almost 50,000 women die from such complications. About 100,000 women survive a hip fracture annually but become at least partially disabled for life. It is estimated that as many as 25 percent of the women who suffer hip fractures must enter a nursing-home or other long-term-care facility.

Aftermath of a Hip Fracture

It is startling to read the stark statistics and learn that each year thousands of women find their quality of life dramatically diminished because of a hip fracture. It can be heartwrenching to read the details of how a hip fracture can steal an individual's mobility and independence and force her from her home. Ellen, an 83-year-old widow, lived alone. She had suffered a fracture of her upper right arm that had not healed well and required a splint. Despite the awkward arm splint she maintained an active independent life and was able to take care of her own needs. One small misstep changed her whole life. Ellen stubbed her toe while climbing some concrete steps at her home and fell, sustaining a fracture to her right hip. The fracture was repaired and, after a short stay in the hospital, Ellen moved to a rehabilitation program to help her regain mobility. Her progress was limited but sufficient to allow her to be discharged from the program, and she returned home. Unfortunately, Ellen was not able to resume her previous lifestyle and required frequent visits from a home-health nurse and more than once-daily visits from a daughter who lived nearby. It soon became obvious that Ellen's plan to return to independent living was not working as she had hoped. This formerly active woman who had so recently been able to care for herself could no longer leave her home without assistance. Within three months of her fracture, Ellen was essentially housebound. Her behavior gradually changed, she developed an abnormal sleep-wake cycle, and in time she gradually became more and more confused. The physician suggested nursing-home care but Ellen and her daughter were reluctant to consider such a move. Unfortunately, Ellen's condition continued to decline and, within four months of her fracture, admission to a nursing home was a necessity, not an option. Ellen's story is typical of thousands of women who lose their independence in a matter of months following a hip fracture.

Unavoidable Risks

A number of conditions put a woman at risk for osteoporosis and the harmful consequences of bone fracture. Perhaps one of the biggest risks is being female. Approximately 1 in 3 women who live to be 90 years old will suffer a hip fracture while only 1 in 6 men who reach 90 will have the same misfortune. Men enjoy a greater degree of protection against osteoporosis because in their early years they naturally develop more bone mass than females. There is also some evidence that men have higher levels of calcitonin, the hormone associated with bone formation. In addition, testosterone protects the bones of men just as estrogen protects those of women. However, men are not faced with a counterpart for menopause and do not experience a swift decline in testosterone. This allows their bone loss to occur more gradually, and accounts for the fact that males lag 20 or more years behind women in developing symptoms of osteoporosis.

Frame size also has a significant impact on a woman's risk for osteoporosis. Petite small-boned women, regardless of body weight, carry the highest risk for osteoporosis. Diminutive size affords limited bone mass at maturity; this contributes to the moderately early age at which small women usually develop osteoporosis. Large-boned women, on the other hand, have significantly greater total bone mass at maturity and usually become fracture-prone later in life.

Some women are at increased risk because they have a grandmother, mother, aunt, or sister who has osteoporosis. Since osteoporosis was not always diagnosed in generations past, some women need to do a little sleuthing to determine their family history. A close female relative who became visibly shorter with age, developed a dowager's hump, or suffered a broken wrist or hip after 45 or 50 years of age presents strong evidence of osteoporosis. If you are not sure whether or not your grandmother shrank with age, a look at the family album may provide important clues concerning osteoporosis in the family tree. However, a lack of osteoporosis in one's family history does not guarantee healthy bones because osteoporosis sometimes appears in families with no past record of the disease.

Skin tone is another indicator of a woman's risk for osteoporosis. The fairer a woman's complexion, the more meager her bone density at maturity. That makes fair-skinned women with ancestors from northern Europe, Britain, Japan, or China more likely to develop osteoporosis. For these women, the rapid loss of bone mass can result in fragile, fracture-prone bones long before the age of 60. Black women, whose ancestry is from more southern latitudes, are protected by high bone mass at maturity. They also tend to produce higher levels of calcitonin. This does not mean that dark-skinned women never get osteoporosis, but the disease usually does not appear until late in life.

An early or premature menopause (before age 40) is another characteristic common among women with osteoporosis. A woman's menopause will probably fall in the same age range as that of her mother, aunts, and older sisters. Premature menopause due to a hysterectomy with oophorectomy can pose an even greater risk for osteoporosis than natural menopause. The threat of osteoporosis related to premature menopause stems from the reduced number of years that estrogen is present to protect against bone loss.

Diabetes mellitus, which may or may not be inherited, also increases the probability of osteoporosis. There are two forms of diabetes. Both affect the body's ability to produce and use insulin properly. *Insulin-dependent diabetes mellitus (IDDM)* usually begins early in life, apparently has a genetic component, and requires insulin to control the disorder. *Noninsulin-dependent diabetes mellitus (NIDDM)* is the more common form of diabetes, and does not generally occur until adulthood. However, many adults are unaware that they have the disease. NIDDM does not seem to be inherited, but instead is influenced by some of the same risks that affect osteoporosis — smoking, obesity, and lack of exercise. Proper diet, weight loss, and medications other than insulin are often sufficient to control NIDDM. Women with diabetes should minimize its effects on their bones by taking appropriate medication and eating a suitable diet outlined by a physician.

Bone-Robbing Drugs

Certain health problems may require one of a number of drugs that stimulate bone loss. Anticonvulsants, furosemide diuretics, heparin, aluminum-containing antacids, steroids, and high doses (more than 3 mg) of thyroid hormone all promote accelerated bone loss. Obviously, the benefit of a medication like an anticonvulsant far outweighs any added risk it may contribute to osteoporosis. When a drug that promotes bone loss is required, ask your doctor for help in maintaining bone mass and strength. A physician may suggest simple exercises and a balanced diet that includes adequate calcium and vitamin D. For many women, hormone replacement therapy may also be advised.

There are alternatives for some bone-robbing drugs that provide equal protection without encouraging bone loss. This is true for some types of diuretics used to treat hypertension. *Furosemide diuretics* allow or promote the loss of body calcium in the urine while *thiazide diuretics* decrease urinary calcium and apparently increase or at least preserve bone density in elderly women. A group of Boston-based researchers assessed the relationship between thiazide use and subsequent hip fractures among postmenopausal women who participated in the Framingham Heart Study and reported their findings in a recent issue of the *Journal of the American Medical Association*. Women who had used thiazide diuretics in the past were not protected from hip fractures, but current or recent users of pure thiazide diuretics were protected and had fewer hip fractures.

Alternative choices are also available for antacid users. Amphojel, Delcid, Di-Gel, Gelusil, Maalox, Mylanta, Riopan, Rolaids, and Simeco are among the brands that contain aluminum, which contributes to calcium loss and can impact on the rate of bone loss. It is usually easy to substitute an aluminum-free antacid like Alka-Seltzer, Alka-2, Bisodol, Citrocarbonate, Eno, Marblen, Percy Medicine, Titralac, or Tums. The calcium contained in some of these guards against bone loss and can serve as part of the required daily calcium intake. The contents of an antacid can be determined by a quick check of the label or by asking a pharmacist.

Habits Can Make a Difference

Physicians and health service agencies continually remind women to control their weight for their health's sake, but when it comes to osteoporosis, thin equals high risk. A low estrogen level is the common link between a slender body and osteoporosis. After menopause, estrogen production by the ovaries is significantly reduced, even though the ovaries and adrenal glands continue to manufacture substantial amounts of androgens that are converted into estrogen. Obese postmenopausal women have a real advantage when it comes to converting androgen into estrogen because they have more fat tissue—the main site for the conversion process. Consequently, the plump enjoy a higher degree of natural bone protection from estrogen than their thin counterparts.

However, this is not a good excuse to pig out with impunity. Obese women have a 3 to 9 times higher risk of developing endometrial cancer than their slender companions and are also at greater risk of cardiovascular disease. The protection offered by excess pounds is a poor trade-off. Estrogen replacement therapy, proper nutrition, and exercise are more effective and healthier ways of reducing the risk of osteoporosis.

Evidence that links the smoking habit to accelerated bone loss and an increased risk of osteoporosis has been available for several years. Scientists compared the bone mass in three groups of women—nonsmokers, women who smoked one-half pack of cigarettes each day, and women who smoked a whole pack each day. During the course of the study, the nonsmokers lost the least amount of bone. Among the smokers, the pack-a-day smokers lost more bone mass than smokers in the half-a-pack-a-day group. The obvious conclusion was that the more a woman smokes, the more bone she loses. Just cutting down on the number of cigarettes smoked each day is helpful. Quitting is better.

Alcohol use also has the potential to promote osteoporosis at least in part because it decreases the intestinal absorption of calcium. When alcohol is present in the body, much of the calcium ingested stays in the intestinal tract and passes with the feces. The body never gets a chance to use this calcium for building bones or for other critical body functions. Some experts suggest that it may be advisable to avoid drinking alcoholic beverages for an hour or more before and after taking a calcium supplement or eating a meal rich in calcium-containing food. Most agree that moderate use of alcohol (two alcoholic drinks each day) may not pose a significant risk of osteoporosis. Scientists do not know at what level alcohol consumption becomes a significant factor in bone loss, but a woman who has one or more other risk factors for developing osteoporosis may wish to limit alcohol use. It is well established that alcoholics have a significantly increased risk for osteoporosis.

A Puzzling Pain

Osteoporosis is truly a silent epidemic that often strikes with no warning signs. Women who add to natural risks by smoking or drinking to excess court disaster. Lauren's story is a traumatic testimony to the effect undiagnosed osteoporosis can have on a woman's quality of life. At age 50, Lauren became increasingly troubled with severe pain in her right chest and abdomen but had suffered no accident or other notable trauma that might account for such pain. She sought help from a number of specialists, but none were able to find the source of her discomfort. The fact that she smoked and had a chronic cough appeared unrelated. Every attempt at diagnosis seemed to end in a blank wall as one medical test after another gave negative results and offered no clue. Having exhausted all the seemingly obvious avenues, the physician scheduled more tests including a colonoscopy to determine if an intestinal problem might be at the root of Lauren's elusive problem.

By this time, the search for relief had dragged on over several months. Lauren's physicians remained hopeful of finding an explanation for her pain, but she grew tired of hurting and began to think the pain might be a manifestation of some psychological problem. The discomfort and the thought that the problem might be in her head led Lauren to heavy drinking. Finally, feeling out of control and suicidal, she appeared at the local hospital emergency room seeking help.

On admission, Lauren's chest pain was noted and chest X rays were ordered. During Lauren's long search for an explanation for her pain, X rays had never been taken because there was no history of a fall or other injury. The X rays revealed the reason for Lauren's pain. The 8th, 9th, and 10th ribs on Lauren's right side had been fractured—apparently rather recently. Fractures somewhat older in appearance were present in the 4th, 5th, 6th, and 7th ribs on the same side! Additional testing confirmed that the fractures were indeed related to a significant loss of bone mass due to osteoporosis. Lauren had added to her natural risk factors for osteoporosis by smoking and excessive drinking. Her ribs were so fragile that the fractures were apparently caused by the minimal trauma of coughing spells related to her smoking. Such fractures are not unusual for women with severe osteoporosis.

Lauren's story is a fairly common one. Many physicians—and women—associate osteoporosis with advanced age. At 50, Lauren did not fit the expected stereotype of a women with severe osteoporosis. As a result of the stereotypic expectations, Lauren's painful condition persisted undiagnosed for an extended period of time. Osteoporosis does not respect youth or age. It is an opportunistic disorder that takes advantage of declining estrogen levels and thrives on self-imposed risks like smoking, excess alcohol use, poor nutrition, and a sedentary lifestyle.

Measuring Bone Density

Evaluating personal risk factors serves as an indicator of a women's chances of suffering from osteoporosis but does not determine her actual bone loss.

A woman at high risk for osteoporosis may wish to have her physician monitor bone density with one of the currently available techniques. Baseline measurements can be made to determine present bone mass followed by additional measurements at periodic intervals to determine the rate of bone loss. *Single-photon absorptiometry* of the wrist and dual photon absorptiometry of the spine can detect losses as small as 1 to 2 percent of bone mass. Another method, quantitative *computerized tomography* (*CT*), is more accurate in detecting early bone loss in the spine but is not widely used because it is expensive and requires exposure to high doses of radiation. X ray can only detect osteoporosis after a minimum of 30 percent of the bone mass is lost.

7

The
Heart
of the
Matter

Women and Heart Disease

Most women shudder when they hear the words "one in nine women," and the fear of breast cancer immediately leaps to mind. Did you know, however, that with the decline in estrogen levels during the years preceding and following menopause the risk of cardiovascular disease meets and exceeds the risk of breast cancer? According to recent statistics from the American Heart Association, one in nine women between the ages of 45 and 64 has some form of cardiovascular disease. After the age of 65, a woman's risk of heart disease jumps to one in three. Each year approximately 2.5 million American women are hospitalized for cardiovascular illness. It is the leading cause of death among women in the United States, killing 500,000 women annually. That means that it accounts for over one-third of all female deaths in this country, which surpasses the death rate for all forms of cancer combined.

Only recently has the medical community clearly appreciated the grave risk that heart disease poses for women, but it is clearly an equal opportunity killer when it comes to the sexes. Each year almost half (247,000) of the 520,000 fatal heart attacks strike women. Data from the Framingham Heart Study were instrumental in establishing the threat of heart disease to women. Set in Framingham, Massachusetts, the study began in 1948 and remains an ongoing endeavor. The project initially included women and men aged 30 to 62 and was designed to study the risk factors for coronary heart disease in a community setting. Analysis of the data show that between the ages of 45 and 54, the incidence of coronary heart disease is three times higher in men than in women. After age 65 the gap begins to narrow and by age 75 the incidence of heart disease is the same in men and women. The age discrepancy between the appearance of heart disease in men and women reflects the protective quality of estrogen on the female cardiovascular system prior to menopause. Young women can and do suffer from heart disease, but as indicated above, heart disease becomes more common as women age. Among the participants in the Framingham Heart Study, postmenopausal women aged 55 and older were at ten times the risk of coronary heart disease as women aged 35 to 54.

Race also influences the risk of heart disease among women. This is reflected in a much higher death rate in black women (181.1 deaths per 100,000 population) than in white women (114.2 deaths per 100,000 population). The reason for this difference is not clear, but may be related to the fact that black women suffer a higher incidence of diabetes, which is a serious risk factor for heart disease. People with a family history of heart disease are also at increased risk and account for over 50 percent of all cases that occur before the age of 55.

Cholesterol Numbers

Over 20 years ago, data from the Framingham Heart Study indicated that participants with low levels of cholesterol in the blood had a low incidence of coronary heart disease. Conversely, people with high levels of cholesterol had a high incidence of coronary heart disease. These and similar findings prompted the medical community to wage war against the high cholesterol levels of Americans. The attention is warranted, because an estimated 65 million Americans have cholesterol levels that are considered too high to be healthy. However, the widespread publicity urging Americans to lower their cholesterol levels has given the false impression that cholesterol is an alien invader, detrimental to the human body. That is far from the truth. Cholesterol is a critical component of cell membranes and a number of hormones including estrogen, progesterone, and testosterone. It is also necessary for the manufacture of bile acids that are important for digestion. Finally, cholesterol plays an integral role in the process that shuttles fats throughout the body. Even though cholesterol is vital to good health, excess cholesterol can clog arteries and increase the risk of cardiovascular disease.

Controlling the amount of cholesterol we eat helps maintain the amount of cholesterol in the blood or total serum cholesterol at a level that is reasonable. Cholesterol levels can be determined by a simple blood test that yields results in milligrams of cholesterol per deciliter of blood (mg/dL). Many physicians and other health professionals frequently omit the units and express cholesterol levels as numeric measurements. The National Cholesterol Education Program, a branch of the National Heart, Lung, and Blood Institute, has established accepted guidelines that recommend a total serum cholesterol of 200 mg/dL or less to minimize the risk of heart disease. About half of all Americans have cholesterol levels in this range.

Some authorities suggest that even readings of 200 mg/dL are too high and recommend that the optimum total cholesterol level is between 150 and 160 mg/dL. This recommendation is based in part on data from the *Multiple Risk Factor Intervention Trial* that was aptly nicknamed Mr. Fit because of the acronym and because the study included only men. The study found that serum cholesterol levels as low as 180 mg/dL are associated with an increased risk of mortality. However, the risk increases steadily above levels of 200 mg/dL, so this value is generally cited as the maximum acceptable level for men and women. Approximately 50 percent of adult Americans have total cholesterol readings well above this range. Some 30 percent have total serum cholesterol levels between 200 mg/dL and 239 mg/dL, which puts them in a borderline-risk area. Another 20 percent of the population has cholesterol levels above 240 mg/dL and are considered at significant risk of heart disease.

Some individuals carry genes for *familial hypercholesterolemia* (inherited high cholesterol) that cause extraordinarily high cholesterol levels. The body of an affected person simply cannot deal properly with cholesterol. This genetic disorder can be responsible for serum cholesterol readings of 1000+ mg/dL, which can only be controlled by medication. In addition to the risks posed by high cholesterol levels, there is now some evidence that a very low total cholesterol level may also have a negative impact on cardiovascular health. A level that strikes a happy medium—higher than 100 mg/dL and lower than 200 mg/dL—is probably best.

Cholesterol is a waxy, fat-like substance, and does not mix in the bloodstream, the body's transport system for nutrients. To overcome this problem, the liver tucks cholesterol and fats into microscopic spheres and wraps each with a water-soluble protein coat that easily dissolves in the bloodstream. These water-soluble *lipoprotein particles* come in different sizes and weights, depending primarily on the ratio of lightweight cholesterol and fat to heavyweight protein each contains. We hear most about *very low density lipoprotein (VLDL), low density lipoprotein (LDL),* and *high density lipoprotein (HDL).* The relative amount of each of these also serves as an indicator of a person's risk for cardiovascular disease.

In 1985, Drs. Michael Brown and Joseph Goldstein earned a Nobel Prize for studies explaining how the body regulates levels of cholesterol and fats. Specifically, they determined the role of VLDLs, LDLs, and HDLs. The process starts in the liver where cholesterol and fat are packaged into very low-density lipoprotein particles that contain a great deal of lightweight cholesterol and fat and only a small amount of heavy protein. The VLDLs travel in the bloodstream to muscle and adipose cells that use fat. These cells have special VLDL receptors that attach to the VLDL particles, extract their fat, and release the particle as a smaller, lighter cholesterol-containing low-density lipoprotein particle or LDL.

About half the LDLs produced return to the liver and are recycled into new VLDLs. The rest deliver their cholesterol load by attaching to LDL receptors on cell surfaces. Drs. Brown and Goldstein found that each cell can regulate the amount of cholesterol that enters by adjusting the number of LDL receptors on its surface. When cholesterol is needed or when only a small amount is available, the cell increases the number of LDL receptors; this is equivalent to increasing the number of doors available to cholesterol. Conversely, when little cholesterol is needed or when cholesterol is plentiful, the cell decreases the number of LDL receptors or eliminates doors and limits the amount of cholesterol that can enter.

In limited numbers, the LDLs play an important role since they carry about 65 percent of the body's cholesterol. Unfortunately, LDLs become a problem if their numbers are large. A diet high in cholesterol and fat prompts the liver to produce more VLDLs to package the excess fat. These VLDLS deliver the surplus fat to storage sites (hips and thighs) where they are transformed into LDLs. The large number of LDLs quickly meet cellular demands for cholesterol. Cells respond to the tremendous number of circulating LDLs by decreasing the number of LDL receptors available. A great many LDLs are left free in the bloodstream with no place to go. Many of these extra LDLs become lodged in the smooth walls of blood vessels where they accumulate and form *atherosclerotic plaques* that grow with the addition of LDLs and cellular debris. This decreases the diameter of the blood vessel, limits blood flow, and increases the risk of coronary heart disease. It is this role of excess LDLs that gives the particles the nickname of "bad cholesterol." Drs. Brown and Goldstein suggest that a high cholesterol/high fat diet creates a *lifestyle-induced deficiency of LDL receptors* that initiates or exacerbates atherosclerosis. The generally acceptable range for LDL is 104 to 130 mg/dL. Values in the lower end of the range are more desirable. Limiting cholesterol and fats in the diet and eliminating smoking can help achieve a lower LDL level. A recent National Institutes of Health report indicated patients with LDL concentrations greater than 150 mg/dL who cannot decrease the level through these methods may require drug therapy.

The concept of an "ideal lipoprotein profile" was recently complicated by findings presented at a meeting of the American Heart Association. Researchers have found that among patients with the same LDL cholesterol levels, some have three times the risk of coronary heart disease because of the genetically determined size of their LDL particles. Patients with the condition have a predominance of small LDL particles that are apparently more prone to produce atherosclerotic plaques. The genetic condition has been found in postmenopausal women, as well as men. The disorder is usually accompanied by triglyceride levels greater than 140 mg/dL and HDL cholesterol levels less than 35 or 40 mg/dL. However, these readings do not provide a positive indicator for the genetic condition. A specific test for the atherosclerosis-susceptibility gene that is an indicator for the disorder will not be available for several years.

As mentioned previously, the liver also packages cholesterol in the form of high-density lipoprotein particles or HDLs that have relatively little light cholesterol and fat and more heavy protein. HDL particles have been nicknamed "good cholesterol" because they can retrieve LDL particles stuck in blood vessel linings and clean up atherosclerotic plaques. However, HDL is limited in the amount of damage it can undo. An HDL level between 35 and 85 mg/dL is satisfactory, but some researchers suggest it be at least 40 to 45 mg/dL. In general, the more HDL present to clear clogged arteries, the better.

Several factors can affect HDL levels. These levels are at their best when ideal weight is maintained (or at least held to less than 20 percent over ideal weight), and regular exercise is part of a lifestyle routine. Women who stop smoking will enjoy a rise in their HDL levels. Estrogen replacement therapy enhances HDL levels of postmenopausal women who otherwise suffer declining HDL readings. There is also some evidence that moderate alcohol consumption (less than 1 ounce/day) may increase levels of HDL, although drinking is not suggested as a therapeutic measure (see Chapter 9).

Considerable evidence indicates that improving HDL is worth the effort. For example, the Helsinki Heart Study evaluated patients who began the study with low HDL levels and high LDL levels. They found that in this group, every 1 percent increase in HDL cholesterol was linked to a 3 percent decrease in heart disease. Only males were included in the Helsinki project, but researchers assume that women who improve their cholesterol levels will realize similar benefits.

The risk of cardiovascular disease is also affected by the triglyceride (fat) level in the blood. High levels of dietary fat are responsible for high triglyceride values that can elevate LDL levels. Triglycerides should range between 30 and 190 mg/dL, but the lower levels are more desirable. Excess alcohol consumption increases triglyceride levels in the blood and should be avoided. This does not mean that abstinence is necessary, but some experts recommend that alcohol intake be limited to one ounce per day.

A recent report from the National Institutes of Health states that the total serum cholesterol value representing the combined levels VLDL, LDL, and HDL is no longer a sufficient indicator of the risk of cardiovascular disease. Many people have acceptable total cholesterol levels, but low HDL or high LDL or triglyceride levels. A true assessment of cardiovascular risk requires knowing the level of each type of cholesterol and how it relates to the total cholesterol level. A risk factor for heart disease can be calculated by dividing the total cholesterol level by the HDL level. As a rule of thumb, a ratio of more than 4.5 indicates that a man is at risk. However, women naturally have higher HDL levels than men, and a ratio of more than 4.0 suggests some risk. Table 1 lists generally accepted risk factors for coronary heart disease. Risks factors for men are included for comparison.

Note that if a woman has a total cholesterol of 200 mg/dL, the maximum recommended, and her HDL is 35 mg/dL, the minimum recommended, her risk factor is 5.7 (200/35 = 5.7). This implies that she is at above average risk of coronary heart disease. It is important to discuss the entire lipid profile with a physician when evaluating personal risk for heart

Table 1.
Risk Factors Determined by Cholesterol Ratio

Women	Men	Risk Factor
3.3	3.4	1/2 average risk
4.4	5.0	average risk
7.1	9.6	2 × average risk
11.0	24.0	3 × average risk

disease. Women at high risk may require medication to control triglyceride and cholesterol levels.

Estrogen's Role

Estrogen plays an important role in maintaining healthy cholesterol levels and a healthy cardiovascular system. Overwhelming evidence indicates that postmenopausal women receiving estrogen replacement therapy have about half the risk of cardiovascular disease as postmenopausal women not using estrogen. Even women with hypertension, diabetes, or a history of stroke are candidates for this therapy. An estimated 25 to 50 percent of the protection is attributed to the positive impact of estrogen on the lipoprotein levels in these women. There is no question that after menopause estrogen replacement increases beneficial HDL levels and decreases detrimental LDL levels. This is an especially advantageous change because the level of LDL commonly rises after menopause, presumably because of loss of estrogen-stimulated LDL receptor activity.

Possibly the most remarkable protection afforded to postmenopausal users of estrogen replacement therapy can be seen in the significant reduction in risk of severe coronary artery disease and stroke. Physicians generally agree that women not receiving estrogen replacement therapy are at about 50 percent greater risk of coronary heart disease than postmenopausal women who are taking estrogen replacement therapy. According to the National Center for Health Statistics, estrogen replacement therapy also decreases the number of strokes in postmenopausal women by up to 31 percent and may reduce deaths from stroke by 63 percent.

Most studies concerning postmenopausal cardiovascular risk documented the protective effects of estrogen alone. Then it was determined that postmenopausal women with a uterus dramatically reduced their risk of endometrial cancer by adding a progestin (progesterone-type drug) to their estrogen therapy. Some experts thought the presence of a progestin might decrease the benefit of estrogen. However, a 1993 report in the *New England Journal of Medicine* found that the use of estrogen combined with progestin appears to produce better HDL, LDL, and triglyceride profiles than those observed in women taking estrogen only. As a matter of fact, users of estrogen alone had higher triglyceride levels than users of estrogen with progestin or women not receiving hormone therapy.

How does estrogen protect the cardiovascular system? Investigators speculate that 50 to 75 percent of the beneficial effect of estrogen on the risk of coronary heart disease comes through avenues other than an effect on cholesterol levels. The presence of estrogen receptors in the myocardium (heart muscle) implies an estrogen influence on the heart itself, although a specific estrogen function has not been determined. Estrogen receptors are also present in the smooth muscles of blood vessel walls where they are known to affect vasodilation (increased blood vessel diameter). How and to what degree protective benefits are realized through the interaction of estrogen with these receptors is not known. A variety of additional mechanisms probably mediate the advantages of estrogen replacement therapy, although none are well understood at present. It appears that estrogen replacement therapy has a beneficial influence on blood pressure, glucose levels, and insulin levels, as well as other factors.

In the face of overwhelming evidence that estrogen replacement therapy affords postmenopausal women significantly decreased risks for cardiovascular diseases, it is amazing that up to two-thirds of the women have discontinued their use of prescribed hormone replacement therapy for various reasons. Women who continue on estrogen replacement therapy are, by definition, compliant women. Studies show they are also more likely to be white, educated, upper-middle class, and lean. Whether this profile makes them naturally more prone to a lower incidence of coronary heart disease is under investigation.

The Ailing Circulatory System

A number of disorders can compromise the function of the heart and blood vessels, but the four most widespread and devastating are hypertension, atherosclerosis, coronary heart disease, and stroke.

Hypertension

Hypertension, commonly referred to as *high blood pressure*, has virtually no symptoms and causes no pain. Yet it is a major risk factor for atherosclerosis, heart attack, stroke, and kidney disease. According to the Joint National Committee on Detection, Evaluation, and Treatment of High Blood Pressure, the number of Americans with high blood pressure has declined by 14 percent in the last 10 years. That is fantastic news, but hypertension continues to overwork the hearts of about 50 million Americans, putting them at great risk for compromised quality of life or death.

Hypertension affects the circulatory system by making the heart work harder. The average adult heart is about the size of a man's fist and weighs only 10 to 14 ounces. Despite its small size, the rhythmic beating of the heart keeps the body's 10 pints of blood in continuous movement through approximately 60,000 miles of blood vessels. The blood carries oxygen, nutrients, hormones, electrolytes, and other substances to the body's cells, and removes carbon dioxide and wastes. The activity level of the heart is incredible—60 to 80 beats each minute, 100,000 beats each day, and 2.5 billion beats in a lifetime. The heart circulates the blood through the body so often that it pumps the equivalent of 2000 gallons of blood each day in an average individual. If that sounds amazing, consider that the heart of an active athlete may pump 4000 gallons of blood in a day.

A person's blood pressure reading indicates how hard the heart is working to pump blood through the body. The reading is composed of two numbers expressed in millimeters of mercury (mm Hg). The first, larger number represents the *systolic pressure* or the maximum pressure in the blood vessels when the heart is contracting. The second, smaller number is the *diastolic pressure* that signifies the residual or constant pressure produced by the blood that remains in the blood vessels when the heart is relaxed. As the heart contracts, it must push or work against the blood that is already in the arteries and veins in order to force more blood into the vessels. The greater the blood pressure in the vessels between heart beats (diastolic blood pressure), the harder the heart has to work to push more blood into those vessels when it contracts.

The normal blood pressure is about 120/80 mm Hg (120 over 80 millimeters of mercury) in a healthy young adult. High blood pressure in an adult is defined as a systolic pressure that is equal to or greater than 140 mm Hg and/or a diastolic pressure that is equal to or greater than 90 mm Hg. The magnitude of the diastolic pressure is sometimes further classified as mild (90 to 104 mm Hg), moderate (105 to 114 mm Hg), or severe (115 mm Hg or higher).

Excess weight and a sedentary lifestyle are primary factors that contribute to high blood pressure. Consequently, weight loss through diet and exercise is often the first step a physician recommends to a hypertensive patient—especially if she is more than 20 percent over her ideal weight. Studies show that *diastolic blood pressure is reduced an average of 6 mm Hg for every 10 pounds of weight lost.* Of course, gaining weight can have the reverse effect. Exercise helps control weight and according to recent studies also helps control blood pressure even when weight loss does not occur. Walking briskly three to five times a week for at least 30 minutes is sufficient to effect a positive change in blood pressure for many people.

Alcohol consumption, salt intake, and smoking are other lifestyle habits that can contribute to high blood pressure. People who regularly drink more than two ounces of hard liquor (or the equivalent) each day usually have an elevated systolic pressure. Excessive salt intake also tends to elevate the diastolic pressure. This is a considerable problem since Americans consume an estimated 3 to 20 times the amount of salt they need. Recently, there has been an increased awareness of the impact of alcohol and salt on cardiovascular health. Americans have responded to the danger and, according to the National Heart, Lung, and Blood Institute, the per capita alcohol consumption fell approximately 12 percent and salt intake was reduced by about 14 percent during the 1980s. Decreased alcohol and salt consumption are no doubt primarily responsible for the fact that the number of people with high blood pressure dropped from 58 million in 1980 to 50 million today.

There is also irrefutable evidence that smoking results in a rapid short-term rise in blood pressure with every cigarette lit. This means the heart must work harder. In addition, the amount of oxygen available to cells is seriously diminished. The long-term effects on hypertension are under study but smoking aggravates many health problems, such as atherosclerosis, which additionally contribute to hypertension. Finally, some data indicate that long-term (over 5 years) use of oral contraceptives may contribute to hypertension in some women. If hypertension develops while taking oral contraceptives, switching to another type of contraception should be considered.

Atherosclerosis

Atherosclerosis or *hardening of the arteries* is widespread among Americans, as well as individuals in many other countries where red meat, dairy products, and other foods containing high levels of animal fat constitute a major portion of the diet. These foods are high in cholesterol and saturated fats that can result in a build-up of fatty deposits on the otherwise smooth blood vessel walls. These deposits clog the blood vessels and limit the flow of blood; this in turn raises the blood pressure. Problems can also arise when tiny blood clots that are normally harmless clog an already restricted blood vessel and stop the flow of blood completely. A blockage of this type is serious anywhere in the body, but in the arteries that supply the heart or brain can cause a heart attack or stroke.

Hypertension and atherosclerosis can set in motion a vicious cycle in which each condition exacerbates the other and both escalate the workload of the heart. In a healthy individual, the blood vessels are somewhat elastic, allowing them to give slightly to accommodate the surge of blood that accompanies each heartbeat. Atherosclerosis decreases the diameter of blood vessels and may also cause them to lose much of their elasticity. This forces the heart muscle to work harder than normal to pump the blood against a higher diastolic pressure and into a smaller, less elastic system. These conditions tend to elevate diastolic pressure and precipitate hypertension; this can then damage blood vessel linings and aggravate atherosclerosis. With extra and very demanding work, the heart muscle becomes more easily fatigued, can be more easily damaged, and has a smaller reserve to draw on. Reserve cardiac power is very important if the body must respond to an unexpected external demand such as danger, fear, anger, or surprise. Atherosclerosis and hypertension are contributing factors to coronary heart disease—the number one cause of death in the United States. They are also major risk factors for stroke.

Coronary Heart Disease

Approximately 5 million Americans currently suffer from *coronary heart disease*. Of these millions, approximately 500,000 die each year—nearly half are women. Coronary heart disease progresses as the tiny arteries that supply the heart muscle, the *coronary arteries*, begin to narrow due to atherosclerosis and decrease blood flow to the cells of the heart muscle. In some cases, an atherosclerotic deposit grows so large it completely blocks the coronary artery. In others, a small blood clot may become lodged in the restricted region of the coronary artery. Either situation can significantly reduce the blood flow to the heart. With insufficient oxygen and nutrients the heart muscle soon becomes weakened and/or damaged. If a coronary artery is completely blocked, nearby heart cells begin to die. This is the beginning of a *heart attack* or *myocardial infarction*. On average, almost three Americans suffer a heart attack every minute of each day, adding up to about one and a half million heart attacks each year.

When a heart attack strikes, the heart can no longer pump an adequate amount of blood to supply the rest of the body. Victims suffer intense pain. More than 80 percent of heart attack victims feel crushing chest pain that is not relieved by rest. In almost 70 percent of the victims, the pain radiates down the left arm or up the neck and jaw. Other symptoms include weakness, sweating, a feeling of impending doom, nausea, and sometimes vomiting.

It is not completely clear why women go undiagnosed for heart attack more frequently than men. It is possible that women and physicians fail to recognize the symptoms when a woman has a heart attack. Once diagnosed, women do not always receive the same care as a man. A study of nearly 5000 heart-attack patients at the University of Washington in Seattle found that only 14 percent of women, compared to 26 percent of men, received clot-busting drugs that can halt a heart attack in progress. Women are also only half as likely to undergo angioplasty, a procedure in which a "balloon" is inserted into a blocked artery to reduce the blockage. Women who do undergo angioplasty have variable results. A study at Duke Medical Center showed that, following angioplasty, arteries closed up again in 46 percent of premenopausal women, 38 percent of postmenopausal women, and 35 percent of men. This data has led researchers to believe that premenopausal women may have a more aggressive form of heart disease. Other reports indicate that by-pass surgery is also less effective in treating women than men. Again, the reason is unclear. It could be that there is an underlying physiological difference between men and women. Others have suggested that some physicians are less adept in dealing with female anatomy. One thing is evident; the evaluation of therapeutic procedures has included men almost exclusively. Women are at equal risk and must be involved in research programs studying heart disease and its treatment.

Risk factors for coronary heart disease include a family history of heart disease, hypertension, atherosclerosis, smoking, obesity, a high-cholesterol and high-fat diet, diabetes, and a sedentary lifestyle. Black women are at greater risk than white women and suffer 22 percent more heart attacks. This is probably related to the fact that the incidence of diabetes (another risk factor) is much higher among black women.

Recent information from the Nurse's Health Study indicate that the use of 1 to 6 aspirin per week decreased a woman's risk of a first myocardial infarction by 25 percent when compared to women who took no aspirin. Similar information has been available for men for some time but studies have only recently investigated the effects of aspirin on women. The data are not yet conclusive, but look promising. Caution is necessary since the use of aspirin may cause gastrointestinal discomfort and bleeding in some women. High doses of aspirin have also been associated with an increased risk of stroke (see below). Reasonable doses, 1 to 6 aspirin per week, may serve as protection from cardiovascular disease for women who are not candidates for estrogen replacement therapy but should be taken only on the advice of a physician.

Stroke

Stroke is the nation's third leading cause of death among women. The incidence of stroke is slightly higher in males, but 61 percent of those who die from stroke are women. Many female stroke victims are postmenopausal women, and dwindling estrogen levels are implicated as a risk factor. Estrogen replacement therapy appears to decrease the incidence of stroke in the postmenopausal age group. However, 10 percent of female stroke victims are under 50 years of age.

About 80 percent of strokes occur when blood vessels supplying the brain become blocked. The blockage may be caused by an atherosclerotic plaque or clot (thrombosis) that forms within a blood vessel or by a clot or foreign body (embolism) that forms in some other part of the body, wanders to the brain, and lodges in a blood vessel. When a stroke occurs, the nerve cells served by the affected artery begin to die from lack of oxygen. Symptoms include dizziness, numbness or weakness in an arm or leg, blurred vision, difficulty speaking, and confusion. Another 15 percent of stroke victims suffer from *hemorrhagic strokes* that have similar symptoms but are due to ruptured blood vessels that cause severe bleeding in the brain. The hemorrhage generally occurs at a spot in a brain artery that has been weakened—usually by hypertension or atherosclerosis. Results from the Framingham Heart Study indicate that hemorrhagic strokes occur most frequently on Monday mornings. Investigators call it "stormy Monday" and are now looking for risk factors and behaviors that might contribute to the Monday morning onset of stroke.

Risks for stroke include family history of stroke, hypertension, smoking, high-fat/high-cholesterol diet, sedentary lifestyle, diabetes, obesity, and extended use of oral contraceptives (especially in older premenopausal women who smoke). Black women suffer 75 percent more strokes than white women. This is also related to the high incidence of diabetes among black women.

Strokes can occur without warning and can have a wide range of effects that sometimes result in a temporary or permanent impairment. The extent and exact nature of debility caused by a stroke vary with the location of the particular nerve cells that are damaged or killed by insufficient oxygen. Each side of the brain controls the function of the other side of the body, therefore the death of cells in a small localized area may result in paralysis of one side of the face or of a single arm or leg. If more cells are involved, one entire side of the body may be affected. The left side of the brain also contains areas associated with speech and language. People with left-brain damage sometimes have difficulty speaking and understanding. Right-brain damage can affect centers that control spatial perceptions and may make judging distance, size, and position difficult. Damage to either side of the brain can result in blindness or hearing loss on the other side of the body and in memory loss or personality changes. In the best-case scenario, most women suffer a decrease in quality of life and many require long-term health care.

Moderate doses of aspirin are sometimes recommended for the prevention of stroke. Aspirin prevents blood platelets from sticking together and presumably lowers the risk of clots. However, according to a 1994 study in the *British Medical Journal* aspirin may cause bleeding in the brain and should not be taken by those at low risk for stroke. Your physician is the best judge and should be consulted before taking aspirin for a prolonged period.

8

Hormone Replacement Therapy

Hormones from the Drug Store

"I'm too old to be young and too young to be old" was the tearful lament of Evelyn Couch in the movie *Fried Green Tomatoes*. Through her sobs, she acknowledged breaking into sweats with her heart pounding, bursting into tears for no reason at all, and having a voracious appetite for candy bars. Chuckling with the wisdom of one who knew the symptoms, Ninny Threadgood offered an explanation and suggested a cure, "Honey, you're going through the change. . . . You get yourself some hormones."

In her middle years, Evelyn was experiencing some of the symptoms of menopause that can be alleviated by *hormone replacement therapy (HRT)* or *estrogen replacement therapy (ERT)*. HRT combines estrogen and a synthetic progesterone and is appropriate for women who have a uterus. ERT provides estrogen alone and is prescribed for women who have had their uterus removed. (HRT is sometimes used as a general term to include both ERT and HRT.) Many women believe that they realize significant benefits from HRT and elect to use it in their peri- and postmenopause years. However, hormone replacement is not for every woman. Before deciding for or against HRT, a woman should recognize the popularized misconceptions about hormone use, consider the potential benefits, and be aware of the side effects and possible drawbacks of the therapy. Then a well-informed individual choice can be made to use hormones after menopause or to explore other avenues of therapy to relieve symptoms, preserve bone mass, and protect the cardiovascular system. The current status of HRT in the minds of women and the medical community can be put into better perspective by knowing a little about the history of the therapy, the background concerning HRT and the cancer scare, and the actual risk of cancer according to the latest scientific data.

HRT and the Cancer Scare

Estrogen has had a relatively short and somewhat turbulent history since it was first described in the early part of this century. The development of drug therapy progressed by leaps and bounds in the first half of this century. Estrogen was produced as an oral contraceptive and also as a replacement therapy for the natural estrogens lost at menopause. Even with all this advancement, the perception of menopause and menopausal women changed very little. Robert Wilson, the well-known proponent of estrogen replacement therapy in the 1960s, referred to menopause as "a galloping catastrophe." Wilson advocated estrogen replacement therapy for post-menopausal women proposing that, "Such women will be much more pleasant to live with and will not become dull and unattractive." Wilson's attitude was typical of the 1960s and even 1970s. The thinking of the medical community at that time was steeped in centuries of misconceptions and misinformation about menopause. Wilson's assessment of menopausal women was not meant to be cruel—it was "modern medicine" in the 1960s.

Estrogen was considered by some to be a silver bullet that could "cure" everything from hot flashes and wrinkles to depression and waning sex drive. Women no doubt did benefit from the estrogen replacement therapy, but it was not the fountain of youth that Wilson and others proclaimed it to be. The reasons for prescribing estrogen replacement therapy in the 1960s may have been flawed, but physicians supported the new treatment with vigor. Premarin, still a widely prescribed form of estrogen, became the fifth most popular drug in the United States, and by 1975, 6 million women were taking it.

With estrogen use at its peak, two independent researchers published articles in *The New England Journal of Medicine* that linked estrogen replacement therapy to an increased risk of endometrial cancer. The use of estrogen replacement therapy plummeted. Today repercussions from those reports have left many women terrified of the threat of cancer. The fear is reflected in the findings of a field study by McKinlay that was described by Dr. Lila Nachtigall in *Obstetrics and Gynecology*. Over 1700 women who had been given a prescription for hormone replacement therapy were surveyed to determine how many women faithfully used the prescribed medication. An amazing 30 percent of the women never filled the prescription, and another 10 percent took the hormones only on an irregular basis. Over half of the women who never filled the prescription or who stopped taking it did so because they were afraid of cancer. Such low compliance may not be a general rule, but the study emphasizes the fact that the fear of cancer is a problem for many women. It is important for a woman to examine all of the facts about the cancer risk before deciding whether or not to take HRT. However, a patient owes it to herself and her physician to express any intentions not to follow the physician's recommendations. The doctor may wish to explore other avenues of therapy if she understands the patient's feelings.

The 1975 investigations demonstrated a somewhat increased incidence of endometrial cancer among women who were receiving a hormone replacement regimen of *unopposed estrogen*, estrogen only with no progesterone. More recent studies confirm that there is indeed an increased risk of endometrial cancer with unopposed estrogen use. However, these studies also show that *endometrial cancer rates are reduced when estrogen is used with a progestin* (synthetic progesterone). For example, principal investigator Dr. Lynda Voight and her coworkers at The Fred Hutchinson Cancer Research Center in Seattle reported that the risk of endometrial cancer among women who had used unopposed estrogen for more than three years was over five times (relative risk 5.7) that of women who had used no hormones. In Dr. Voight's study as well as other follow-up studies, it was concluded that women who took estrogen but also received a progestin for 10 or more days each month have little or no excess risk (relative risk 1.1) of endometrial cancer compared with women who took no hormones at all. It is interesting to note that women who use oral contraceptives that contain higher doses of estrogen and progestin have an even lower risk of endometrial cancer—about half that of women not on the Pill. The greater reduction of endometrial cancer risk is related to the the higher concentrations of the hormones present in the contraceptives.

How does estrogen alone increase the risk of endometrial cancer? Estrogen in moderately low doses can encourage the growth of the endometrium or uterine lining. Unrestricted, the growth of the endometrium can lead to precancerous or even cancerous changes in cell structure. During a normal menstrual cycle this does not occur because progesterone arrests the growth of the endometrium, promotes differentiation of endometrial glands, and initiates sloughing of the endometrium (the menstrual flow). When a progestin is included in an oral contraceptive or added to hormone replacement therapy, the action is much the same, and the endometrium is not permitted to grow unchecked under the influence of estrogen. It seems that controlling the growth of the endometrium is the key to virtually eliminating the threat of endometrial cancer. The current consensus in the medical community is that women receiving hormone replacement therapy should be given both estrogen and a progestin if they have a uterus. There is, however, no mandate that requires estrogen and progestin be prescribed together for women with a uterus. Naturally, women who have had a hysterectomy do not have the concern of endometrial cancer and need not take a progestin with estrogen. The data strongly indicate that, properly prescribed, HRT poses no significant risk for endometrial cancer.

Whether or not a woman is taking hormone replacement therapy, the risk of dying from endometrial cancer is not great. The death rate is about 3000 women per year. Compare this to approximately 50,000 women who die each year from complications related to hip and other fractures and another 250,000 who die of heart attacks. These risks are greatly diminished for women who use hormone replacement therapy. One group of researchers determined that the combined risk of death from endometrial cancer, hip fracture, and heart disease was 17.5 percent for a 50-year-old woman receiving no hormone treatment. On the other hand, a 50-year-old woman receiving estrogen replacement therapy had only a 10 percent risk for death from one of the three. The difference was due to the reduced risk of hip fracture and heart disease for a woman on estrogen replacement therapy.

While investigators were busy trying to determine the actual risk of endometrial cancer for women on HRT, a second cancer demon reared its ugly head. The new concern was whether or not estrogen, with or without progestin, increased the risk of breast cancer. A number of studies designed to address this question have produced varying results. Most investigators conclude that there is virtually no increased risk of breast cancer due to hormone replacement therapy. Other studies have reported a marginal risk (often less than 1 percent). The very few studies that report a greater risk of breast cancer (more than 1 percent) related to hormone replacement therapy have been criticized for flaws in experimental design. The general consensus seems to be that the majority of investigations have failed to prove a significantly increased risk of breast cancer for "the average woman." HRT is not advised for women with a history of breast cancer or for women who have other factors that place them at high risk for breast cancer. For most women, however, there presently seems to be no specific argument that supports an increased risk of breast cancer due to HRT and, therefore, no reason to change from a recommended therapy.

HRT – The Benefits

Estrogen replacement therapy offers a host of additional benefits that improve the quality of life. ERT reduces and in many cases virtually eliminates a long list of menopause symptoms that includes hot flashes, night sweats, sleeplessness, insomnia, vaginal dryness and atrophy, painful sexual intercourse, dizziness, headache, forgetfulness, and irritability. HRT also improves feelings of well-being and has a positive influence on mood. Improvement of some symptoms apparently results from correcting others. For example, estrogen usually eliminates or drastically decreases night sweats; this in turn improves the quality of sleep, which reduces irritability.

The data supporting the long-term use of hormone replacement therapy to maintain and/or increase bone mass in postmenopausal women is also strong. A recently published study followed 2800 women in a free-living community for 6 years. The study clearly documents the devastation that can be caused by hip fracture. Among the participants in the study, 120 had hip fractures and of these 18 percent died. Those who survived suffered drastic changes in their lifestyles. Before their fractures, 86 percent of the women could dress themselves, but less than 50 percent could do so after their fracture. Mobility was also dramatically reduced for many. Before their fracture, 75 percent of the women could walk across a room, but only 15 percent could accomplish this seemingly small but critical feat afterward. Similarly, 41 percent of the women could walk half a mile prior to their fracture, but only 6 percent regained that type of mobility after recovery. The women who lost mobility experienced a dramatic change in the status of their independence and their quality of life. They required nursing-home care or another form of long-term care that provided assistance. Inestimable benefit can be derived by using hormone replacement therapy to reduce the risk of hip fracture and the potential complications that often follow.

Adequate calcium, vitamin D, and exercise are important supporting procedures, but ERT is the only effective way to combat osteoporosis in postmenopausal women. One long-term study tracked women for 10 years following oophorectomy. The group taking estrogen replacement therapy experienced little bone loss during the 10-year period, while the women taking a placebo suffered significant bone loss. These results are typical of a number of studies published over the past several years. There seems to be no doubt that estrogen replacement therapy preserves and in some cases increases bone mass. As a result, a woman's potential for fracture and the difficulties that follow are significantly reduced.

A hip fracture can be devastating and may lead to death, but coronary disease poses an even greater threat to postmenopausal women. It is estimated that a woman between 50 and 94 years of age has a 31 percent risk of death from coronary disease and a much lower 2.8 percent risk of death from hip fracture complications, 2.8 percent risk of death from breast cancer, and 0.7 percent risk of death from endometrial cancer. This does not decrease the gravity of the threat of death from the three latter conditions. It does put into perspective the enormity of the threat of heart disease to postmenopausal women. Recent evidence that estrogen protects against the development of cardiovascular disease in women may provide a method of reducing the risks. Results of several studies have been reviewed, and many researchers within the medical community now believe that current estrogen users have a risk of coronary heart disease that is 50 percent lower than that of nonusers.

A number of physicians believe that the strong evidence pointing to a substantial reduction in coronary heart disease risk is sufficient reason to recommend HRT for patients. Estrogen impacts many biological actions that could influence the risk of coronary heart disease including lipid metabolism, carbohydrate metabolism, blood clotting factors, and blood pressure. Researchers speculate that there may be additional effects of estrogen on the heart muscle or coronary arteries since these tissues have estrogen receptors.

Misconceptions and Side Effects

It is important to remember that HRT is not a cure-all. Wrinkles, grey hair, and other age-related changes will still occur. Estrogen may enhance the quality of the skin and can certainly enhance the quality of life, keeping one young at heart. Many women use hormone replacement therapy with no problems. Others, however, may encounter some side effects.

Being past menopause and on hormone replacement therapy does not necessarily mean that a woman is free of a type of menstrual flow. Many women are given estrogen for 28 days with a progestin added during the last 10 or 12 days. The progestin promotes sloughing of any endometrial growth encouraged by the estrogen and results in what is termed *withdrawal bleeding*. The name reflects the fact that bleeding occurs when progestin is withdrawn or stopped. The flow, however, is similar to the premenopausal menstrual flow. Continuing the routine of monthly periods is annoying to some women and often causes them to discontinue their therapy.

Recently, more physicians have begun to prescribe continuous daily use of both an estrogen and a progestin that minimizes cyclic withdrawal bleeding. *Breakthrough bleeding* does sometimes occur, but seems to decrease in frequency after several months of the combined therapy. There has been some concern that progestin might decrease some of the beneficial effects of estrogen and has caused some physicians to be reluctant to prescribe the combined estrogen and progestin regimen. To date, however, there is no strong evidence to support this concern. Some physicians reason that it is desirable for women to enjoy at least some of the benefits of estrogen even if progestin is found to compromise its effects. The two other obvious options are to omit estrogen replacement completely or to withhold progestin and increase the risk of endometrial cancer. Neither approach seems acceptable.

Weight gain is another commonly listed side effect of hormone replacement therapy. This is considered by some researchers to be a misconception. In a long-term study, headed by Dr. Lila Nachtigall, coauthor of *Estrogen*, women on similar diets had identical weight gain after 10 years regardless of whether they had taken estrogen or a placebo. Estrogen can influence where weight is added, encouraging fat deposits on the hips and thighs in the typical female pattern. There is a tendency for edema or water retention in some women taking hormone replacement therapy. This type of bloating can be very uncomfortable, but is not actually a weight gain. Edema should be discussed with a physician. According to Dr. Nachtigall, swelling and bloating can often be remedied by taking vitamin B$_6$ which acts as a mild diuretic.

Nausea and breast tenderness are other side effects occasionally experienced. These too should be discussed with a physician. Simple changes can sometimes eliminate an annoying problem. For example, nausea can sometimes be relieved by switching from oral estrogen to a transdermal patch. Whatever the difficulty, a physician should be willing to listen and attempt to make alterations that will make hormone replacement therapy a pleasant experience.

How Much Is Enough?

Approximately 14 percent of American postmenopausal women are currently receiving hormones to replace those their bodies produce in meager amounts after menopause. Nearly 3 percent of these women use HRT and about 11 percent receive ERT. Both pills and patches are considered effective in relieving transient symptoms like hot flashes, preventing osteoporosis, and providing protection against the risk of cardiovascular disease. The length of hormone treatment depends on a woman's symptoms, risks, and her physician's experience and opinions. Some authorities believe that estrogen should be taken primarily in the few years of the perimenopause when transient symptoms are most troublesome. Another group of physicians recommend estrogen replacement therapy for 10 years, while still others prescribe it for the lifetime of their postmenopausal patients to protect against osteoporosis and cardiovascular disease.

The duration of treatment is not the only variable. Estrogen, progestins, and estrogen-testosterone combinations all come in a variety of formulations (molecular variations) and in a range of doses. A number of studies have determined that a dose of 0.625 mg to 1.25 mg conjugated estrogen (see below) or the equivalent is sufficient to alleviate menopausal symptoms for most women. Unfortunately, some physicians believe this guideline is carved in stone and prescribe this dosage for all patients. While 0.625 mg of conjugated estrogen adequately controls menopausal symptoms for many women, it is not adequate for all women. This poses a problem for women who find their physician reluctant to explore other possibilities in order to find the correct dose for each patient.

Karen was in such an unfortunate situation. Fibroid tumors and pelvic pain prompted Karen to have a total hysterectomy with the removal of both ovaries at age 45. Her physician quickly prescribed 1.25 mg conjugated estrogen in an effort to prevent the transient symptoms of menopause that rapidly appear after the removal of the ovaries. The estrogen adequately protected Karen from some symptoms of menopause like hot flashes, but she was bothered by vaginal dryness, irritability, and complexion changes including acne. Her physician ignored her complaints and pointed out that she was receiving ERT. Four years later, in exasperation and frustration, Karen sought out another physician who listened to her problems. The new doctor checked Karen's FSH levels and found them to be considerably elevated at 76.8 MIU/ml. Karen's distressing symptoms subsided shortly after her ERT dosage was increased to 2.5 mg conjugated estrogen. Karen's experience was unfortunate but not uncommon. Women are not all alike. Finding the right hormone therapy for an individual may require exploring different dosages, formulations, or routes of administration.

Estrogen

The estrogens available for clinical use are the *natural estrogens* (conjugated equine estrogen, esterified estrogens, 17β-estradiol, estradiol valerate, estrone, estrone sulfate, micronized 17β-estradiol, and others), *synthetic steroids* (ethinyl estradiol, methyl ethinyl estradiol or mestranol, and quinestrol), and *synthetic nonsteroids* (chlorotrianisene, dienestrol, and diethylstilbestrol). The synthetic nonsteroids are not commonly prescribed even though they are potent estrogens. One of them, diethylstilbestrol (DES), was used in the 1950s to ward off potential miscarriages, but was later associated with birth abnormalities in the daughters of women who took DES during pregnancy.

Pills

Estrogen-containing tablets designed for oral administration are probably the most popular form of natural and synthetic estrogens. Tablets containing *conjugated estrogens* have been used since 1941 and are still the most widely prescribed form of oral ERT. Conjugated estrogens are modified (partially metabolized) in structure but are capable of attaching to estrogen receptors and initiating function. They are considered natural estrogens because they are obtained from the urine of pregnant mares—a natural source. They contain a mixture of forms of estrogens including *estrone*, the second most prevalent human estrogen, and *equilin*, an estrogen found in horses but not in humans. No detrimental effects have been directly attributed to the presence of equilin, but some physicians have expressed concern about its presence. Recent studies do show that estrone and other naturally occurring human estrogens are broken down and eliminated from the body in 24 to 36 hours. Equilin, on the other hand, remains in the human body for 30+ days after ERT usage has ended. Whether or not the extended presence of equilin has any significant effects on human health remains to be seen. The only brand of conjugated estrogens currently available is *Premarin*, which is distributed by Ayerst Laboratories in five different oral dosages. Premarin also comes as a vaginal cream and in combination with methyltestosterone, an androgen (see below).

Estradiol is the most potent of the estrogens and the most abundant natural form of estrogen during a woman's reproductive years. Estradiol was not widely prescribed in early years, because the natural form is not readily soluble in water, which makes it poorly absorbed by the gastrointestinal tract. To overcome this problem, some pharmaceutical companies produce tablets that contain slightly modified forms of estradiol that are more readily absorbed by the gastrointestinal tract but still retain estrogen activity in the body. *Estinyl* (ethinyl estradiol) by Schering-Plough and *Estrovis* (quinestrol) by Parke-Davis are two such products. Recently, Mead Johnson Laboratories developed *Estrace*, a micronized form of estradiol, that can also be efficiently absorbed and used by the body.

Other companies have taken another tack. Abbott Laboratories distributes *Ogen* tablets and Ortho Laboratories markets *Ortho-est*. These two products contain *estropipate*, a natural estrogenic substance prepared from estrone, the less potent form of estrogen. In the dosages available, the effects are comparable to those of estradiol and conjugated estrogens.

Patches

Estrogen, or any other drug, taken orally passes directly from the stomach or intestinal tract to the liver. The liver serves as a sort of clearing house before the estrogen is distributed throughout the rest of the body by the circulatory system. In the liver, the estrogen molecule may be changed or partially metabolized to another form. This process can affect the strength of the drug and accounts, in part, for the fact that different forms of estrogens are available in different dosages. It is sometimes desirable to eliminate the "first pass" of a drug through the liver.

Ciba Pharmaceuticals manufactures an estradiol-containing skin patch (*Estraderm*) that circumvents the liver first pass by allowing the hormone to directly enter the general circulation. Estrogen is distributed throughout the body before it is altered by the liver, thus providing a more uniform level of drug than is available from oral sources.

Estraderm was originally approved by the FDA for the treatment of menopausal symptoms because investigators were able to show that the newer estradiol-containing transdermal patches are as effective as estrogen in tablet form for decreasing menopause symptoms. One such study was reported by Dr. Veronica Ravnikar of Harvard Medical School who demonstrated the effectiveness of transdermal patches in controlling hot flashes in postmenopausal women. Either remedy, pill or patch, may require a little patience for optimum results. Some relief from symptoms is usually noticed within a short time since the level of estrogen in the bloodstream rises soon after the initiation of estrogen replacement therapy. The incidence of hot flashes and related symptoms continues to gradually decrease. Maximum benefits are reached after a period of several days or a few weeks.

Transdermal estrogen-containing patches have recently received approval for use in the prevention of osteoporosis. This approval is the result of several studies that documented the efficiency of Estraderm in preventing bone loss in postmenopausal women. For example, a recent Mayo Clinic study evaluated the use of the patch and a placebo in 98 postmenopausal women over the age of 40. At the end of the 2-year trial, bone density remained stable in Estraderm users. Women who received a placebo averaged 6.4 percent bone loss in the spine and 4.9 percent bone loss in the wrist.

Evidence confirming the efficiency of transdermal patches in controlling menopause symptoms and osteoporosis has given women and their physicians more flexibility in selecting a method of treatment. Some women seem to get greater benefit from transdermally delivered estradiol. Others simply prefer changing patches twice a week rather than contending with a daily regimen of pills. The patch adheres somewhat like a bandaid and is usually applied to the lower trunk on the abdomen or buttocks. A minor skin irritation at the patch site occurs occasionally, but moving the patch and applying it to another dry area of skin sometimes remedies this difficulty.

Vaginal Cream

Estrogen is also available in cream-form that can be applied vaginally using a slender applicator. Available products contain conjugated estrogens (*Premarin* by Ayerst), 17β-estradiol (*Estrace* by Mead Johnson), estropipate (*Ogen* by Abbott), estrone (*Oestrilin* and *Neo Estrone*), or the synthetic estrogen dienestrol (*Ortho Dienestrol* by Ortho and *Estragard* by Solvay). Estrogen very readily passes across the vaginal membranes and into the circulatory system which can significantly increase the level of circulating estrogen in the body. Vaginal creams are usually intended to control symptoms confined to the urino-genital region because it is difficult to control the precise dose when estrogen is administered in this manner.

Estrogen-containing creams were originally intended to alleviate vaginal atrophy and painful intercourse when no or few other menopausal symptoms were present. Recently, Drs. Raul Raz and Walter Stamm evaluated their use in the prevention of recurrent urinary tract infections. A group of 93 postmenopausal women with a history of urinary tract infections were divided into two groups and vaginal cultures and pH were monitored. During the course of the study, one group of women used estrogen-containing vaginal cream each night for two weeks and then twice weekly for eight months. The control group followed the same schedule but used a placebo cream. The majority of women in the estrogen group remained free of urinary tract infections over the eight-month course of the experiment. Furthermore, beneficial lactobacilli returned in these women and the vaginal pH dropped from 5.5 to 3.8. At the same time, the presence of pathogenic bacterial colonies declined from 67 percent to 31 percent. The placebo group experienced no significant changes during the course of the study. The investigators concluded that intravaginal use of estrogen-containing cream prevents recurrent urinary tract infections in postmenopausal women. There is evidence from other studies that estrogen replacement therapy in pill form also prevents these infections.

Estrogen Injections

Estrogen preparations in an oil carrier are available for injection by a physician. Some of the available products contain estradiol valerate (*Delestrogen* by Squibb and *Estraval* by Reid-Rowell), estradiol cypionate (*Depo-Estradiol* by Upjohn), and conjugated estrogens (*Premarin IV* by Ayerst). Estrogen by injection is used more slowly by the body and has a longer-lasting effect that can be a great advantage. However, if the physician wishes to terminate treatment with the estrogen, there is no quick withdrawal method. Estrogen in the body must continue to be slowly metabolized until it is depleted.

Progesterone and Progestins

The ovary produces natural progesterone that is important in controlling different processes during the menstrual cycle and pregnancy. *Progesterone* is the term reserved for natural progesterone made by the body or for products that contain molecules identical to the natural progesterone molecule. Until recently it was primarily available only in vaginal suppositories prepared independently by pharmacists. A micronized form of progesterone, *Uterogestin*, has been developed by Key/LaSalle. *Progestins* or *progestagens* are progesterone-like drugs that are derived from progesterone or testosterone. These differ somewhat in structure from natural progesterone but have effects similar to the natural hormone. Progestins are used for HRT primarily because progesterone, even in micronized form, is very poorly absorbed and causes sleepiness. It is recommended that women who still have a uterus and are receiving estrogen also receive progesterone or a progestin to decrease the risk of endometrial cancer. Women who do not have a uterus can take unopposed estrogen. A number of companies produce progestins in tablet form for HRT. These are more commonly prescribed than progesterone suppositories because they are more practical.

Medroxyprogesterone acetate is derived from progesterone and is the most widely used progestin. It is available in a range of doses (2.5 mg, 5 mg, and 10 mg) as *Provera* by Upjohn. Medroxyprogesterone acetate in 10-mg tablets only are available as *Amen* by Carnick and *Curretab* by Reid-Rowell. Norethindrone (*Micronor* by Ortho) and norgestrel (*Overette* by Ayerst) are two of the more commonly used progestins that are derived from testosterone.

Estrogens and Androgens

Tablets that contain a combination of estrogen and testosterone are also available. This formulation is prescribed when menopause symptoms include a decline in libido. Some women experience growth of facial and body hair and develop other masculine traits when using a regimen that includes testosterone. Women with these reactions may elect to eliminate the androgen and use a product containing only some form of estrogen. Combination products contain *methyltestosterone* (a synthetic derivative of testosterone) and conjugated estrogens (*Premarin with methyltestosterone* by Ayerst) or methyltestosterone and esterified estrogens (*Estratest* and *Estratest H.S.* by Solvay Pharmaceuticals).

9

You Are
What You
Eat

Too Many Pounds

For years, scientists have been trying to convince us that what we eat—or don't eat—directly affects our health. This is certainly true during the years following menopause when women face increasingly high risks for cardiovascular disease, osteoporosis, and some forms of cancer. These risks can be substantially magnified by dietary factors. For example, excess weight and a diet high in cholesterol, fat, and salt elevates the risk of cardiovascular disease. Excess use of alcohol and caffeine appears to increase the probability for both cardiovascular disease and osteoporosis. While moderation is the key for some foods, it is necessary to maintain adequate amounts of others. A diet with inadequate calcium and/or vitamin D augments the risk of osteoporosis. Proof is accumulating that appropriate amounts of vitamins A and E and beta-carotene may fend off damage associated with aging and some cancers common in the years following postmenopause.

The importance of eating healthy during the years before and after the menopause transition should not be surprising considering the cumulative impact of poor nutrition on the health and life expectancy of individuals of all ages. Dr. J. Michael McGinnis of the U.S. Department of Health and Human Services and Dr. William Foege of the Carter Presidential Center estimate that the combination of dietary factors and sedentary activity patterns are responsible for at least 300,000 deaths each year. Their recent report in the *Journal of the American Medical Association* indicates that several studies have associated dietary factors or sedentary lifestyles with 22 to 30 percent of cardiovascular deaths, 20 to 60 percent of fatal cancers, and 30 percent of diabetes mellitus deaths. These startling statistics do not take into account the contribution of poor diet on a woman's risk for atherosclerosis, hypertension, heart attack, stroke, osteoporosis, diabetes, and some forms of cancer when death is not a consequence. Poor nutrition often goes hand-in-hand with obesity; this further increases the risk for all these diseases and diminishes the quality of health in general.

Body weight does get the attention of many Americans whether or not they are concerned about a healthy diet. About 62 out of every 100 Americans consider themselves overweight, but the Agricultural Extension Service at the University of Tennessee reports that only about 25 out of every 100 people are really overweight. Medically, a person is classified as obese if she is 20 percent above the ideal weight for a woman of her height. However, the concept of being overweight is influenced by the eye of the beholder. Each women has an idealized picture of her body, and personal preferences may be much more stringent than medical guidelines. A woman may be obese in her own mind if she adds an extra 15 or 20 pounds. However, most of us have a little more than a 20-pound leeway before being considered obese by medical standards. For example, a woman who has an ideal weight of 100 pounds has to tip the scales at 120 pounds before she is considered obese. The rest of us who have higher ideal weights can add more than 20 pounds before being considered obese.

There is no doubt that the American concept of "healthy weight" is changing. The Departments of Agriculture and Health and Human Services no longer publish separate weight charts for men and women. Instead, they have combined goals for the sexes and allow a range of 30 pounds or more at each height. Weights at the upper end of each range are generally, but not exclusively, intended for men. The new chart now has recommended weights for people aged 19 to 34 and a second set of values for individuals 35 and over. Those in the 35 and over bracket get a break; the top limit of each weight range is pushed up by 16 pounds. These weight ranges are somewhat relaxed, because the health risks associated with carrying a few added pounds may diminish as one ages. Still, being within a 30-pound weight range leaves a lot of flexibility for a woman who is trying to determine if she is at a healthy weight. Does a person at the top of her accepted weight range need to consider losing weight to maintain her quality of health and reduce the risk of weight-related health problems that become more prevalent following menopause? Weight charts do not give a very clear cut answer to this question.

Maintaining an appropriate weight is so important that doctors are now evaluating body parameters like body mass index and waist-to-hip measurements to predict a "healthy-body size." The body mass index (BMI) uses both height and weight measurements to arrive at a figure that reflects whether a person is at risk of weight-related health problems like elevated cholesterol levels, high blood pressure, heart disease, and non-insulin-dependent diabetes.

BMI is determined by multiplying a person's weight in pounds by 700, dividing that answer by height in inches, then dividing again by height in inches:

$$(weight \times 700)/height/height = BMI$$

For a 150-pound women who is 5′6″ (66″) tall, the calculation would be:

$$(150 \text{ lbs} \times 700)/66″/66″ = 24 \text{ BMI}$$

The overall risk of developing heart disease is very low to low for a person with a BMI value of 25 or less. A BMI of 24 puts the woman in this example at low risk for heart disease due to her weight. In fact, a value under 25 is considered healthy or desirable for most people, but smokers are an exception. Although often thin, smokers are at very high risk for cancer (especially lung cancer), chronic lung disease, cardiovascular disease, and poor general health. A BMI of 25 to 30 reflects a person who is mildly to moderately overweight and has a low to moderate risk of developing heart disease or other weight-related problems. Those with a BMI value over 30 are considered genuinely overweight and are definitely at increased risk for weight-related health problems including a moderate-to-very-high risk of heart disease.

Another parameter, the *waist-circumference-to-hip-circumference ratio*, is used to predict the risk of several diseases. This measurement takes into account the fact that the location of extra pounds can influence disease risk. Researchers think that the weight carried in the abdominal region may pose a potentially greater health risk than weight carried below the waist. Some individuals, especially women, concentrate extra pounds around the hips and buttocks. After menopause, however, women sometimes "lose" their waistline as they add pounds. In general, men tend to add extra pounds at the waistline.

The waist-to-hip ratio is determined by measuring the waist at its smallest circumference and dividing that by the measurement of the hips at its biggest circumference. Studies have shown a possible link between abdominal fat and insulin resistance (a precursor to diabetes) and hypertension, and even general mortality. Risks for weight-related diseases increase for women with a ratio of more than .80 and for men with a ratio of over .95. Men's propensity for a spare tire naturally gives them a higher ratio than women.

The ratio of waist-to-hip is a better measure of mortality risk than BMI in older women according to Dr. Aaron R. Folsom, associate professor of epidemiology at the University of Minnesota. He and colleagues followed BMI and waist-hip circumference ratios of 41,837 Iowa women aged 55 to 69 over a 5-year period. They found that a 0.15 unit increase in the waist-to-hip circumference ratio (adding weight at the waistline) was associated with a 60 percent greater risk of mortality. In comparison, the BMI measurements showed higher mortality rates among the leanest women as well as the most obese women. The data were controlled for age, BMI, smoking, education level, marital status, estrogen use, and alcohol use. Dr. Folsom recommends that hip-to-waist ratios be charted over time to assess the risk of mortality and to track the changing risk of mortality due to weight-related health problems.

Other risk factors need to be considered when assessing risk as a function of BMI or waist-to-hip ratio. For example, as mentioned above, smoking changes everything. A woman's BMI and waist-to-hip ratio may indicate that she is in a low-risk category, but if she smokes, her risk is actually very high. Similarly, one must consider risk factors like age, sex, sedentary life-style, high blood pressure, elevated cholesterol level, low HDL level, heart disease, diabetes, and a family history of disease. A healthy weight can help control some of these risks, like high blood pressure and cholesterol levels, but it does not eliminate all risks. On the other hand, having risks in addition to excess pounds emphasizes the importance of weight loss to improve health and decrease the overall risk of health problems.

Dieting—Good or Bad?

A great many people wish to lose weight to improve their health, their appearance, or both. In 1991, more than 8 million Americans spent $30 billion on weight-loss programs. The number of pounds lost per person varied widely, but experts estimate that the average participant spent $10 to $40 per pound of weight lost. The 1993 June issue of *Consumer Reports* collected information from 95,000 readers concerning their weight-loss attempts during the three preceding years. About 19,000 of these readers had used one of five commercial diet programs (*Weight Watchers, Jenny Craig, Physicians Weight Loss, Diet Center, and Nutri/System*). The survey found that people do lose weight on these programs, although the majority gain most of it back within two years. About 25 percent of the people in the *Consumer Reports* study had kept most of their weight off at the end of two years. This is a much higher success rate than other studies have reported.

It is a fact that as many as 95 percent of people who go on reduced-calorie diets do lose weight only to gain it back again within the two-year period following the diet. Researchers have found that losing weight only to gain it back again or yo-yo dieting may be just as bad from a health standpoint as being overweight in the first place. A recent assessment of data from the Framingham Heart Study found that people whose weight fluctuated frequently or by many pounds had a 50 percent higher risk of heart disease than those whose weight remained stable.

A Plan You Can Live With

If being moderately overweight may not greatly increase a woman's risk of health problems, and yo-yo dieting seems to jeopardize longevity, what are the reasonable options? It may not be necessary or even a good idea to "go on a diet." A woman is often more successful in promoting good health if she sets goals for a healthy life-style that include a nutritious diet with foods she likes and an exercise program with activities she enjoys. A good plan is one a woman can live with for the rest of her life, and the life span is getting longer. The quality of life as a woman passes each birthday is directly related to her diet and activity level. Because nutrition is so vital, everyone should be informed about the foods they eat and how those foods can affect their health.

The Cholesterol Facts

The body uses cholesterol to manufacture sex hormones and cell membranes and to help transport fats. From a nutritional standpoint, it is not necessary to include any cholesterol in your diet, because the liver is able to produce all of the cholesterol the body needs to supply these essential functions. This isn't very practical, however, since cholesterol, which is produced only by animals, is present in all meat, poultry, fish, and dairy products. The goal, therefore, is to keep cholesterol intake at a level the body can handle without overloading the system and increasing the risk of cardiovascular disease.

Experts recommend an intake far below the 500 to 600 milligrams of cholesterol the average American consumes daily. The American Heart Association recommends a sliding scale for determining cholesterol intake. They suggest 100 milligrams of cholesterol per 1000 calories eaten with a maximum amount of 300 milligrams of cholesterol per day. For example, a woman with a daily calorie requirement of 1500 calories should not exceed 150 milligrams of cholesterol each day.

The amount of cholesterol is included in the nutritional values of ingredients on product labels, but don't be confused by advertising claims of low cholesterol, light, or lite on the front of a product. The use of these terms is now regulated by food labeling laws, but check the nutrition panel for the actual cholesterol value. New food labeling laws that went into effect July 1994 require that all processed foods (like soups and hot dogs) carry precise nutritional information including cholesterol content. Distributors of raw, single ingredient products like meat and poultry may choose to provide nutritional information on each package, or it may be available in other forms like store posters.

Trimming Fat the Easy Way

Like cholesterol, fat is essential to human life, but in excess, it too is a major risk factor for cardiovascular diseases. The evidence that decreasing dietary fat appreciably reduces the risk of coronary heart disease is overwhelming. Yet the average American persists with a diet that is 37 percent fat. For the average person, that is approximately equivalent to eating one stick of butter every day!

The American Heart Association, National Research Council, American

Diabetes Association, and other groups recommend that no more than 30 percent of a day's calories come from fat. Since food tables and manufacturers usually give fat content in grams, it is necessary to calculate dietary fat intake in grams. This can be done by multiplying the number of daily calories by 30 percent and dividing the answer by 9 (the number of calories in one gram of fat). The following calculation would apply to a woman who eats 1500 calories per day.

$$1500 \text{ calories } \times .30 = 450 \text{ calories from fat}$$

$$450 \text{ calories}/ 9 \text{ calories per gram } = 50 \text{ grams of fat}$$

Women who have a history of heart disease or who are at high risk for heart disease will probably be cautioned by their doctors to limit their fat intake to 20 or even 10 percent of total calories and should follow their doctor's recommendations about counting calories, grams of fat, and milligrams of cholesterol.

Counting calories and calculating grams of fat can be a pretty daunting undertaking. That is precisely why many Americans give up or never begin a war against fat. There is an easier way to cut the fat that can be quite effective. Simply substitute low-fat ingredients for their high-fat equivalents. Researchers at Pennsylvania State University calculated that switching from high-fat products like whole milk and butter to their low-fat counterparts could decrease a woman's fat intake from an average 37 percent to 23 percent of her calories. Women volunteers at the University of Illinois at Chicago actually tried such a switch and decreased their fat calories even more than the estimated amount. They reduced their fat intake from 37 percent to 20 percent of their total calories and lost 4 to 5 pounds during the 20-week experiment.

A similar investigation at Cornell University in Ithaca, New York, used two groups of volunteers to see what would happen if the same menus were prepared with different ingredients. One group of participants got low-fat versions of food in which fat calories made up 20 to 25 percent of the total calories. The second group got the same dishes prepared in the customary manner with 35 to 40 percent of the total calories coming from fat. At the end of the 11-week study, individuals in the low-fat group had lost an average of 6.7 pounds—twice as much as those in the high-fat group. The low-fat group members were very satisfied with the reduced-fat versions of stir-fry chicken, oatmeal cookies, blueberry muffins, and other conventional dishes. They had cut out a lot of fat and calories without decreasing the quantity of food they ate. Switching to low-fat products can obviously be quite effective in controlling fat in the diet and fat on the hips. It is helpful, however, to know a few basic facts about fat.

Fat Facts

There are two main types of fats, *saturated fats* and *unsaturated fats*. Both are primarily made of chains of carbon atoms, but they differ in the number of hydrogen atoms attached to the carbons.

Saturated Fats

Saturated fats have hydrogen atoms attached to every available site on each carbon atom—the carbon atoms are *saturated with hydrogens*. Most saturated fats are solid at room temperature; the fat in bacon is a good example of a typical saturated fat. Since animals produce only saturated fats, these fats are present in meats, butter, cheese, and other dairy products from animal sources. A few tropical plants also make saturated fats that are present in products like coconut oil, palm oil, and palm kernel oil.

Health professionals discourage getting too many calories from foods containing saturated fats, because they are the most detrimental to cholesterol levels. Saturated fats raise total serum cholesterol levels and LDL levels and are strongly associated with an increased risk for coronary heart disease. Foods high in saturated fats also contain cholesterol, an additional insult to the body's cholesterol levels.

Unsaturated Fats

Unsaturated fats have fewer hydrogen atoms than saturated fats—the carbon atoms are *unsaturated*. *Polyunsaturated fats* lack hydrogen atoms at several (poly) carbon bonds while *monounsaturated fats* lack hydrogen atoms at only one (mono) carbon bond. These fats come from plant sources, are generally liquid at room temperature, and are the primary ingredients in most cooking oils. Corn oil, safflower oil, and other vegetable oils are polyunsaturated fats, and olive oil and canola oil are monounsaturated fats. Poly- and monounsaturated fats reduce total serum cholesterol and LDL levels and are considered preferable to saturated fats for this reason. Polyunsaturated fats also tend to lower HDL levels. Even with this in mind, the consensus is to replace saturated fats with unsaturated fats and to use monounsaturated fats when there is a reasonable choice between a poly- and a monounsaturated product.

Oils are the same in that they all contain 126 calories and 14 grams of fat per tablespoon. The only difference is in the amount of saturated, polyunsaturated, and monounsaturated fat in the different products. As mentioned, plants cannot make cholesterol, so none of the plant oils contain it. The Food and Drug Administration instructed Mazola, Heart Beat, and Crisco oils to remove the "no cholesterol" claim from their advertising, because it perhaps carried the implication that these products are "good for the heart" since they do not contain cholesterol. There seems to be the further implication that some oils have cholesterol.

Plant oils like corn or safflower oil are used to make margarine as a substitute for butter. Margarine is, of course, low in saturated fat and contains no cholesterol, making it an excellent substitute for butter, which is high in both saturated fat and cholesterol. However, manufacturers of margarine do one more thing to complicate the issue of choosing fats. To make a product that is solid, and to improve consumer acceptance, the vegetable oils are put through a process called *hydrogenation*, which adds hydrogen atoms to unsaturated sites. In general, the greater the degree of hydrogenation, the harder or more solid the oil becomes. For example, tub margarines are less hydrogenated than stick margarines. This process has been criticized because it raises the level of saturated fats. However, one of the saturated fats in stick margarines containing partially hydrogenated corn, safflower, or soybean oil is stearic acid which does not raise blood cholesterol.

A more recent and probably more important criticism of hydrogenation is that it changes the structure of the fat molecules in the oils from their natural *cis configuration* to a *trans configuration*. The change is a bit analogous to changing the configuration of a folding lawn chair from open to closed. The open configuration allows a person to sit in the chair, but the closed configuration does not. The functionality depends on the configuration of the chair, even though the structural components of the chair never change. Similarly, the functionality of a molecule may change depending on whether it is in its *cis* or *trans* configuration even though its components are constant.

Two recent Dutch studies indicate that fat molecules in the *trans* configuration raise blood cholesterol levels. According to Dr. Virgil Brown, president of the American Heart Association and professor of medicine at Emory University, more studies are needed to evaluate the impact of *trans* fatty acids on cholesterol levels. The *cis* versus *trans* controversy will probably continue for some time. In the interim, it might be wise to use tub margarines that are less hydrogenated and contain fewer *trans* fatty acids than stick margarines.

Omega-3 Polyunsaturated Fats

The *omega-3 polyunsaturated fatty acids* present in fish oil are another source of fat associated with a reduced risk of coronary heart disease. For example, researchers evaluated heart disease rates among Eskimo populations with diets consisting largely of fish containing high levels of omega-3 oils. The Eskimo cholesterol and triglyceride levels were generally low, but omega-3 fatty acids seem to primarily affect three other factors. First, omega-3 fatty acids appear to reduce the "stickiness" of platelets, resulting in decreased clotting times and diminishing the risk of blood clots. Second, fish oil seems to function in a manner that makes blood vessel walls very smooth, thus decreasing the risk of atherosclerotic plaque formation. Finally, omega-3 fatty acids are reported to enhance the production of prostaglandins that inhibit inflammation. The inclusion of fatty fishes like swordfish and salmon in the diet provides a good source of omega-3 fatty acids. Most physicians recommend natural sources of fish oil and caution against the use of fish oil capsules that have not been adequately studied.

Fiber

Lowering fat and cholesterol intake is not the only way to control cholesterol levels. Foods high in water-soluble fiber help maintain desirable cholesterol levels by reducing the amount of cholesterol absorbed in the intestines. Fruits, dried beans, peas, barley, rice, bran, psyllium, and oat cereals are good sources of water-soluble fiber. Researchers from the Chicago Center for Clinical Research, a division of the Department of Medicine of Rush-Presbyterian-St.Luke's Medical Center in Chicago documented the beneficial effects of dietary fiber in a 1991 issue of the *Journal of the American Medical Association*. A group of female and male volunteers, aged 30 to 65, who had elevated levels of LDL cholesterol were randomly assigned to three groups. The daily diets of volunteers in each group contained measured amounts of oatmeal, oat bran, or farina (control substance that is not high in soluble fiber). At the end of six weeks, the farina control group had no change in cholesterol level. The oatmeal and oat bran groups realized at least a 10 percent reduction in LDL cholesterol. The benefits require two to three ounces (about one-half cup) of oatmeal or oat bran in the daily diet. In this study, oat bran was somewhat more efficient at lowering LDL levels than oatmeal.

This and similar studies have been criticized for factors perceived as flaws in experimental design or interpretation and because a limited number of participants were involved. Still, the consensus seems to be that foods high in soluble fiber tend to lower LDL cholesterol levels. Although oatmeal and oat bran were used for experimental purposes, the other sources of soluble fiber mentioned above can also be included in the diet to promote lower LDL levels. Additional benefits may be gained from high-fiber diets since they are also associated with a lower incidence of breast and colon cancer.

Salt and Hypertension

Doctors have two cardinal rules for women with hypertension, a condition that is more common after menopause. Hypertensive women are told to lose excess weight and to limit their sodium intake. Small amounts of sodium, a mineral in table salt, are absolutely essential for good health. However, in excess, it can promote hypertension because it causes body tissues, including blood, to retain extra water. Blood vessels are forced to accommodate the larger-than-necessary volume of blood; this then elevates the blood pressure. Decreasing salt intake allows the body to reduce the blood volume and helps hypertensive patients lower blood-pressure readings.

Authorities estimate that an average diet contains 6000 mg or more of sodium on a daily basis. Physicians usually recommend that hypertensive patients restrict their sodium intake to 2000 mg per day, which is actually quite a bit of salt. As a guideline, consider that a teaspoon of table salt contains 2500 mg of sodium. It is essential for women with high blood pressure to control their sodium intake, but it is also wise for women with normal blood pressure readings to keep their salt intake at a reasonable level. A daily intake in the range of 3000 mg is recommended by many physicians.

The biggest challenge in controlling salt intake comes from the large amount of sodium included in many processed foods. For example, tomato juice usually contains about 600 mg of sodium in a 6-ounce glass. The only recourse for someone trying to control sodium intake is to read product labels carefully when purchasing processed foods. Using fresh foods greatly simplifies the task of monitoring salt intake.

The U.S. Public Health Service report "Healthy People 2000" contains three specific objectives that encourage the general population to reduce salt intake. The Public Health Service would like to increase the number of people who purchase low-sodium foods, who cook with less salt, and who do not use salt at the table. Following these general guidelines should keep most women with normal blood pressure at a reasonable sodium intake.

Antioxidants and Free Radicals

Vitamins E and C and beta carotene (a precursor of vitamin A) have long been acknowledged as important nutrients. Now they are being viewed in a new light. These nutrients are believed to protect the body against the ravages of *free radicals*, highly active substances formed as by-products of food metabolism. A number of researchers now attribute many of the processes of aging to the effects of free-radical damage and find the compounds especially harmful to cell membranes. Scientists also speculate that free-radical damage may intensify the threat of cardiovascular diseases and some cancers for which postmenopausal women are at high risk.

One of the biggest concerns is evidence that links free-radical damage to an increased risk of atherosclerosis. Current hypotheses suggest that free radicals oxidize LDL, changing it to a form that is much more likely to form atherosclerotic plaques. Others suggest that free radicals also damage blood vessel walls and create sites that encourage atherosclerotic plaque formation. Regardless of the precise mechanism, free radicals definitely appear to play some role in the progression of atherosclerotic damage and increase the risk of coronary heart disease.

LDL particles carry Vitamin E, a potent antioxidant that increases the resistance of LDL to oxidation. Researchers from Harvard recently published two very large studies, one in women and one in men, providing evidence that the use of large doses of vitamin E supplements is associated with a significantly decreased risk of coronary heart disease. The number of participants was huge, 80,000 women and almost 40,000 men, who were followed for eight and four years respectively. Both studies indicated that taking at least 100 IU (international units) of vitamin E daily reduced the risk of cardiovascular disease. However, researchers caution that these findings are from prospective studies and only indicate that more research is needed. Most authorities suggest that large doses of vitamin E are not yet warranted and advise people to wait until large-scale clinical trials have been completed.

Another large prospective study from Harvard evaluated the effect of vitamins C, E, and A on the risks of breast cancer. Large doses of vitamins C and E did not appear to lower the risk of breast cancer among the women in this study. Women with diets low in vitamin A may benefit from a supplement. Be cautioned that the investigators noted the possibility of an increased risk of breast cancer for some women. Evidence suggests that antioxidants may play a role in curbing other diseases. For example, vitamins E and C may retard the formation of cataracts, and beta carotene has been implicated in the prevention of some cancers.

Research has not yet confirmed the impact of a daily multivitamin and mineral supplement on potential free-radical damage. Scientists are disturbed by the fact that many Americans have a vitamin and mineral intake that is far below the *Recommended Daily Allowance* (RDA) set by the National Academy of Sciences. This fact alone may justify taking a daily multiple vitamin, even though their usefulness in limiting free radical damage is still under investigation. It is interesting to note that 8 of 10 medical professionals who were recently polled by the *Medical Tribune* regularly take antioxidant supplements.

Calcium and Vitamin D

During the peri- and postmenopause years, adequate calcium and vitamin D become increasingly important to maintain bone strength and fight osteoporosis. A conference held at the National Institutes of Health (NIH) estimated that the average adult diet contains 450 mg to 550 mg (milligrams) of calcium each day. This is only about half of the 1000 mg Recommended Daily Allowance (RDA) for adults. Calcium is very important to the bone health of women who have passed menopause. These women fall into a special category and have a RDA of 1500 mg calcium — or about three times as much as the average adult consumes. However, osteoporosis is such a widespread problem among women that most experts, including those at the NIH conference, suggest that women increase their calcium intake to 1500 mg per day long before menopause.

It is possible to get 1500 mg of calcium per day from the food you eat, but it is not always easy. Some of the foods highest in calcium are milk (300 mg per cup), cottage cheese (320 mg per 12 ounces), ice cream (190 mg per cup), and spinach (200 mg per cup). Many women choose to take a daily calcium supplement to meet the RDA rather than keep track of their dietary intake of calcium. Calcium supplements are readily available and reasonably priced. Generally, calcium doses up to 2000 mg pose no problem. However, large doses of calcium have been associated with kidney stone formation, so women with a history of kidney stones should consult a physician before taking a calcium supplement.

Vitamin D is another nutrient essential to strong bones because it assists in the absorption of calcium from the intestines. Rather recently, scientists determined that vitamin D is not a vitamin (a complex organic compound required in small amounts in the diet). Instead, it is a steroid hormone that can be produced by the body. Skin contains a precursor that can be converted into vitamin D by exposure to the ultraviolet rays in sunlight. The body's total vitamin D requirement can be met by skin production alone with adequate exposure to sunlight. While this method of meeting vitamin D requirements is possible, it can present a problem. Busy schedules, bad weather, and seasonal changes in the day length can combine to limit sunlight exposure and curtail vitamin-D production. Elderly people who are housebound or institutionalized may find it impossible to rely on sunlight exposure for adequate vitamin D production.

The difficulty in getting enough vitamin D from sunlight was emphasized by a recent study at the U.S. Department of Agriculture Human Nutrition Research Center on Aging in Boston. Investigators found that postmenopausal women living in northern climates were losing bone in the winter. Women in an experimental group took calcium (800 mg) and vitamin D (400 IU) supplements while women in the control group took a calcium supplement but relied on exposure to sunlight for their supply of vitamin D. Women in the experimental group lost half the amount of spinal bone in the winter as a control group of women who did not make enough vitamin D due to limited sunlight exposure in the cold climates.

Vitamin D is present in some foods like fish, liver, and vitamin-fortified milk, but assuring adequate amounts may best be done by taking a supplement. Many calcium supplements include vitamin D, which is probably the most convenient and reliable way to get the required combination of calcium and vitamin D. Regardless of the route, the RDA of vitamin D is 400 IU (international units). Daily doses of 400 IU of vitamin D should not be exceeded, because long-term use of higher doses can have toxic effects on the body.

The French Paradox

Women who enjoy a glass of wine with dinner may be interested in recent reports that suggest moderate wine drinking may have a positive impact on some cardiovascular conditions for which menopausal women are at high risk. However, excessive alcohol use may contribute to an increased risk of cardiovascular disease and definitely exacerbates bone loss associated with osteoporosis. Attention was first drawn to the possible benefits of moderate amounts of wine by studies that linked French wine-drinking habits with a low incidence of heart disease. As a people, the French begin drinking a glass or two of red wine with meals at a very early age. Each day, at least one meal is usually large, heavy, and loaded with cholesterol and fat. Even fruits and vegetables are sometimes accompanied by rich fat- and cholesterol-laden sauces. Yet there is a low incidence of heart disease among French people who combine high-cholesterol and high-fat meals with one or two glasses of red wine. Some researchers have suggested that the red wine "counteracts" the effects of a high-cholesterol diet and provides the French with the low level of cardiovascular disease that they enjoy. It is important to note that in France the rates of alcohol-related diseases are among the highest in the world.

Recently, American researchers studied a similar group of people in California who regularly enjoyed a few glasses of red or white wine with their meals. The findings were much like those in France. Surprisingly, the white-wine drinkers in the group (mostly the women) had an even lower incidence of cardiovascular disease than the red-wine drinkers. The investigators were quick to point out that most of the participants in the study were health-conscious individuals who watched what they ate and exercised regularly. These factors may play a significant role in the cardiovascular health enjoyed by the wine drinkers in the study.

Data continue to accumulate concerning the effects of one or two alcoholic drinks a day (one drink equals 12 oz beer, 5 oz wine, or 1.5 oz

80-proof spirits). Two separate studies, one by the American Cancer Society and another by researchers at the Kaiser Permanente Medical Center in Oakland, California, gathered data on the relationship of alcohol and heart disease in men and women. Both studies reported that a moderate alcohol intake has an apparent protective effect on coronary heart disease. Women who drank occasionally or had one drink a day (up to two drinks/day in the Kaiser Permanente study) were less likely to die of coronary heart disease than women who did not drink at all. A similar study was conducted at the Harvard School of Public Health and reported in a 1991 issue of *Lancet*. This group found that males who drank the equivalent of one or two glasses of wine a day had a 26 percent reduction in heart disease compared with those who drank no alcohol. The authors attributed the results to alcohol's ability to raise HDL cholesterol levels and also to its tendency to make platelets "less sticky" and, therefore, reduce the likelihood of blood clots.

Not all of the news is positive. The Harvard study, as well as many others, found that higher levels of alcohol consumption promoted cirrhosis of the liver and increased blood pressure. The risk for some types of cancer may also increase with alcohol consumption. A 1987 report in the *New England Journal of Medicine* suggested that women who had the equivalent of a single drink each day had a higher risk of breast cancer than nondrinkers. Other studies have failed to confirm an increased risk of breast cancer with such moderate alcohol consumption. However, the American Cancer Society does report that the risk of breast cancer increases at higher levels of alcohol use. Women who had one to four drinks per day were about 20 percent more likely to have breast cancer than nondrinkers. Above that level of alcohol consumption, risks really jumped. Women in this study who had five drinks a day were at an 89 percent higher risk of breast cancer than nondrinkers.

Alcohol is known to have other deleterious effects on women's health. Drinking has been shown to decrease the absorption of calcium by the intestines. Most of the calcium passes through the intestinal tract and leaves with the feces. The body never has the opportunity to use the lost calcium. With this in mind, it seems wise to avoid alcohol for at least an hour before and after taking a calcium supplement or eating calcium-rich foods. Much research remains to be done. For example, it is known that alcoholics are at high risk for osteoporosis, but at what level alcohol consumption becomes a significant factor in bone loss is not clear.

Coffee, Tea, and Cola

The love affair with coffee and other caffeine-containing beverages is centuries old, and most of the adult population still consumes some form of caffeine every day. Coffee starts the morning of 130 million Americans, who by day's end have downed 400 million cups. Then there are all the other sources of caffeine—notably tea, soft drinks, and chocolate—but coffee supplies over 80 percent of caffeine in the Western diet. The millions who consume caffeinated beverages every day should find it helpful to understand how caffeine affects the body and how it may increase the risk of cardiovascular disease and osteoporosis—two big health threats for postmenopausal women.

The effects of caffeine are no secret. Caffeine is a stimulant that is often consumed to fend off drowsiness, sometimes to the point of insomnia. Too much coffee can lead to heartburn, headache, irritability, dizziness, diarrhea, and trembling hands. Excesses are even said to turn simple addition and subtraction problems into a challenge. These side effects may be partially responsible for the trend among Americans to drink less coffee. The national average peaked at 4.2 cups each day in 1962, but is now down to 3.4 cups a day.

Coffee and other forms of caffeine can have a special impact on women. Caffeine causes the body to excrete more calcium in the urine, thus robbing the body of part of its calcium supply and increasing the risk of osteoporosis. The Framingham Study addressed the effects of using caffeine over a 12-year-period and found that a daily cup of coffee increased the risk of hip fracture by 69 percent! The amount of calcium in the diet was not considered. However, Dr. Elizabeth Barrett-Connor headed a team from the University of California at San Diego that did evaluate the relationship of milk consumption on lifetime coffee use and bone density in 980 white women aged 50 to 98. These women were participants in the Rancho Bernardo Heart and Chronic Disease Study. The results, published in a 1994 issue of the *Journal of the American Medical Association*, showed that women who drank a lifetime equivalent of 2 cups of caffeinated coffee each day experienced a decrease in bone density in the hip and spine *unless* the coffee was supplemented with a daily glass of milk. These data underscore the already overwhelming evidence supporting the importance of an adequate lifetime supply of calcium.

Caffeine also appears to affect the risk of heart disease, but the findings are not clear-cut. Dr. Andrea LaCroix, assistant professor of epidemiology at the University of Washington, studied the relationship between coffee consumption and the risk of heart disease in 1130 men, and published her findings in the *New England Journal of Medicine* in 1986. She found that men who drank five or more cups of coffee a day were 2.5 times more likely to have heart disease than men who drank no coffee. Two more recent studies, one done at Boston University and another at Johns Hopkins University, also found that men who drink five or more cups of coffee each day doubled their risk of heart disease.

In the face of what seems positive proof that caffeine contributes to heart disease, other investigations provide contradictory evidence. For example, Dr. Meir Stampfer, associate professor at the Harvard School of Public Health, observed no increased risk of heart disease among 45,000 men aged 40 to 75 who drank four or more cups of coffee a day. Similarly, coffee drinkers who participated in the Framingham Heart Study did not appear to have an increased risk of heart disease.

Explaining the discrepancies is not easy. It has been observed that coffee drinkers also tend to smoke, have high-fat diets, and sedentary lifestyles. Some authorities suggest that these factors, and not coffee consumption alone, may be responsible for the increased risk of heart disease reported in some studies.

The debate over the effects of decaffeinated versus caffeinated coffee muddies the water even more. Dr. Stampfer's work indicates that men who drink four or more cups of decaffeinated coffee each day may be at increased risk of heart disease when compared to caffeinated-coffee drinkers. Other studies report that decaffeinated coffee causes a rise in LDL cholesterol levels and seem to substantiate such a link. However, a study from Stanford University observed increased cholesterol levels when decaffeinated coffee was made from robusta beans. Cholesterol levels were not affected by decaffeinated coffee made from more costly arabica beans.

Clearly, pinning down the health-risks due to coffee consumption is an area that needs additional investigation, especially since currently available data apply almost exclusively to men. What are coffee lovers to do in the meantime? Be moderate. The implied increased risk of heart disease applied only to those men who drank five or more cups of coffee each day. So for most women, it probably is not necessary to completely give up caffeine, but it may be wise to take a calcium supplement and consider limiting daily consumption to one or two servings of coffee, tea, or cola.

10

Survival
of the
Fittest

Exercise and the Quality of Life

Since 1985, about 25 million Americans have started exercising for the first time. Even with this upsurge in activity, in 1992, the National Center for Health Statistics linked 23 percent of the deaths from the leading chronic diseases to sedentary lifestyles. High blood pressure, heart disease, stroke, colon cancer, and diabetes mellitus are among the biggest health risks associated with lack of exercise. The first three are also major risks associated with the postmenopause years. Osteoporosis, another post-menopause threat, is also exacerbated by lack of exercise. While lack of exercise can be devastating, the major benefits of exercise are attainable through minimal efforts—lifting small weights and walking regularly.

If you think you are too busy, too tired, too achy, too fat, too frail, or too old to start exercising, you're probably wrong. The President's Council on Physical Fitness and Sports surveyed 1018 Americans to find out why so many adults, an estimated 60 percent, are sedentary. The Council found that most sedentary Americans do have time for physical fitness—they just don't think they do. Sixty-four percent of the people polled said they would like to exercise more but had less than 10 hours of leisure time each week. The Council did not agree, since 84 percent of the respondents spent at least 3 hours each week watching television, time the Council thought people could use for exercise if they really wanted to improve their fitness.

Starting an exercise program at an early age is best, but beginning an exercise program at any age is better than *sitting* and thinking about exercising or *sitting* and thinking it is too late to start. Claire Willi was swaybacked and sedentary when she attended her first dance class at age 70. At age 99, she was participating in two or three classes a day and taking a two- or three-hour walk in Central Park—rain, shine, or snow. She could do more at 99 than she could at 70 when she felt like "an old lady."

Claire's activities at 99 emphasize two dividends of exercise that women may not think about until later in life. Regular exercise enhances a woman's *quality of life* and allows her to maintain her *independence* in her senior years. These may not seem big concerns if you are now near menopause. The fact is, quality of life and independence in later years should be especially important to you now. It is generally accepted that a woman who is healthy on her 50th birthday will probably live to be 92 years old and perhaps older.

Eighty or ninety may seem old, but, relatively speaking, it is not quite as old as it used to be. Fifteen years ago aging was considered a disease according to Dr. Gene D. Cohen, acting director of the National Institute on Aging. Furthermore, there was no known therapy for the disease of aging. People aged and, as they did, many lost energy, agility, strength, and stamina. A 1981 study in the *American Journal of Public Health* evaluated physical strength among a group of aging women and men. These researchers found that by age 75 nearly two-thirds of the sedentary women could not lift a weight of more than 10 pounds. Almost one-third of these women could not stand unassisted for 15 minutes and almost half could not crouch. Fewer of the 75 year-old sedentary men who were evaluated were equally impaired, but many were. Among the men, nearly one-third could not lift a 10-pound weight, one-quarter could not stand for 15 minutes, and one-third could not crouch. Images of this degree of impairment are what many of us associate with the ages of 80 and beyond. A sad scenario, but it doesn't have to continue or be repeated.

Muscle weakness can result from a number of factors including chronic illness, sedentary lifestyle, nutritional deficiencies, and even aging. However, it is sometimes reversible and many individuals who have lost function can regain a substantial amount of strength. Dr. Maria Fiatarone, of the U.S. Department of Agriculture's Human Nutrition Research Center on Aging at Tufts University in Boston, has demonstrated that the body has amazing powers. She worked with a group of 10 nursing-home patients ranging in age from 86 to 96 years. Of the ten, eight had a history of falls and seven used a cane or a walker. Under Dr. Fiatarone's supervision, the members of the study group lifted small weights three times a week for 10 or 20 minutes. After eight weeks, all the seniors had more than doubled their strength. Two 90-year-old members of the group were even able to get rid of their canes. Another man could get out of his chair without help for the first time in a long while. According to Dr. Fiatarone, seniors don't lose the ability to pick up a 10-pound weight because they are old—they lose that ability because they are out of practice. Sad to say, after the experiment was completed, the nursing home residents slipped back into their inactive TV-watching habits and within a few weeks had lost one-third of the strength they had gained. In a 1994 issue of the *Journal of the American Medical Association*, Dr. Fiatarone and colleagues reported that resistance exercises for the legs done 3 times a week for 10 weeks significantly improved muscle strength in a group of men and women with an average age of 87. Four participants who used a walker prior to the study needed only a cane after the 10 weeks of exercise. A control group of participants did placebo activities including walking, calesthentics while seated, board games, concerts, crafts, and group discussions. As one might anticipate, these activities did not increase the strength of the volunteers. In fact, one person who had used a cane lost ground and required a walker after the study. It is encouraging that the participants who exercised and gained strength were also able to get around with greater ease and increased their overall level of activity.

It is an unfortunate fact that health benefits from exercising cannot be stored to be borrowed against at a later time. Fitness depends on continued regular exercise and a healthy life style in the young as well as the not so young. Regular exercise maintains strength and also increases longevity. Dr. Ralph Paffenbarger, epidemiologist at Stanford University, and his associates studied the relationship between regular exercise and longevity in a group of more than 10,000 Harvard alumni over an 11- to 15-year period. Participants who took part in moderate-intensity sports activities throughout the study period, or who took up sports during the study, had a 23 to 29 percent lower risk of dying from any cause than men who never participated in sports. Similarly, a 16-year Norwegian study of over 1000 middle-aged men reported that the higher the level of physical fitness, the lower the risk of death from cardiovascular disease and all other causes.

In similar investigations, Dr. Paffenbarger found that exercise actually increased longevity among the subjects in the study group. The amount of time added to one's lifespan depended on the age when regular exercise began, but even study participants who started exercising between the ages of 75 and 79 years realized a number of extra months of life. A weekly energy expenditure of 2000 calories resulted in the greatest effect and added as much as 2 to 3 hours of longevity for every hour exercised.

Keeping Pounds Off

Weight can only be lost if a woman burns more calories by exercising than she consumes by eating. When the body needs extra calories, it first depletes the relatively small reserves of glycogen stored in the liver and muscle cells. Then, stored fat molecules are broken down to meet energy demands, and weight is lost. It sounds simple, but in practice losing weight can be very difficult. The body actually has mechanisms that protect against serious weight loss. Each individual's appetite for food and his or her normal energy level maintain a *set point* of body weight. A low-calorie diet—especially one with less than 1200 calories—triggers mechanisms that slow the *basal metabolism* or rate at which calories are burned and makes weight loss more difficult. Since the system tends to preserve weight at its set point, animals are said to "defend" against weight changes. Scientists do not know exactly how the system works, but they believe that increased activity is very important, if not critical, in changing the set point. Over a period of time, exercise combined with a moderate decrease in food nudges the set point to a new lower level.

How much exercise does it take to change the set point? No one knows for certain, but 3500 calories must be burned or exercised away to lose each pound of fat. The more calories an activity uses, the greater the potential to lose weight. Therefore, resting—the principal activity of couch potatoes—burns about 1.1 calories per minute, which does not make a major contribution to weight loss. For example, it takes about 6 hours and 30 minutes to "rest away" a 470-calorie cheeseburger, 2 hours and 32 minutes to "rest off" a 185-calorie slice of pepperoni pizza, and about one hour to "relax away" a 70-calorie apple. What about something a little more physical? Running burns about 14.7 calories per minute (depending on speed), which would consume the calories from the cheeseburger in 32 minutes, the pizza in 12 minutes, and the apple in 5 minutes. That's quite an improvement, but not many people take up a running program and stick to it long term. Walking is an activity that strikes a happy medium between resting and running. A stroll at 3 mph can wipe out the cheeseburger in 1 hour and 28 minutes, the pizza in about 35 minutes, and the apple in 13 minutes. A brisker walk at 4.5 mph would cut these times even more. The cheeseburger would "disappear from the hips" in 1 hour and 4 minutes, the pizza in 25 minutes, and the apple in about 10 minutes. Whatever type of exercise is chosen, it should be one that you like and can imagine yourself continuing for the rest of your life.

As people age, they tend to lose muscle tissue and this presents an additional challenge to someone wishing to stay fit and keep the fat off. Dr. Maria Fiatarone estimates that most people lose 20 to 30 percent of their muscle tissue during their lifetimes, beginning in their forties. According to some authorities, women characteristically trade 7 pounds of muscle for 14 pounds of fat as they age. Strength can go with the muscle, and unwanted weight comes with the fat. In addition, muscle burns calories more rapidly than fatty tissue so some of the efficient calorie-burning machinery is lost with the muscle. Researchers at the Human Nutrition Research Center on Aging recently reported that as people age, inactivity contributes to more excess body fat than overeating.

The importance of exercise was made clear by a research group at Baylor College of Medicine in Houston who compared the effects of diet and exercise on weight loss. The study included three groups: a diet-only group that ate a lean 1200 calorie diet each day but followed no fitness program; a diet-plus-exercise group that combined diet with brisk walking; and an exercise-only group that followed a brisk walking routine but no special diet. In the early part of the study, the dieters lost the most weight followed by the diet-exercisers. The exercise group lost the least. When researchers checked the groups after two years, they found that those in the diet and diet-exercise groups had gained back all of their weight. Volunteers in the exercise group had kept weight off and had continued to exercise and lose weight during the two years that followed the initial program. This reinforces the findings of most studies that evaluate the effectiveness of diets. Within two years of ending a "low-calorie" diet program, the majority of dieters have gained back at least most of what they lost. There is a good chance people feel deprived of favorite foods and/or just get tired of counting the calories in every single bite they eat.

Exercise and Your Heart

Weight control is an asset to good health because excess weight is a risk factor for atherosclerosis, hypertension, heart disease, diabetes, and other diseases that are prevalent in the postmenopausal years. Research findings concerning the favorable effect of exercise on heart health are overwhelming. According to the American Heart Association, a number of scientific studies have documented the fact that inactive people are at 1 ½ to 2 times greater risk of having a heart attack than physically active people. The risk doesn't stop there. The chances of dying immediately after a heart attack are 3 times greater for inactive individuals as for active people. In addition to the 500,000 who die of heart attacks annually, many of the one million heart attack survivors are faced with a decreased quality of life. Exercising can improve cardiovascular health and lower the grim statistics of heart attack.

Major improvements do not take very long. Patricia Porcelli's experience is a good example. Her story recently appeared in an article in *Walking*. Patricia did not have a problem with hypertension until she was 56 years old, when she had gained about 30 pounds and was under stress from illnesses in her family. Suddenly, her blood pressure was 155/90. Her family history was an added concern. Her sister had a stroke at age 41 and her mother had a heart attack in her early 60s. Patricia responded to a newspaper advertisement for people with mild hypertension to take part in a research program at Duke University. The project headed by psychologist James Blumenthal was designed to determine if aerobic exercise could reduce mild hypertension. Patricia was in a group designated to walk, jog, bike, and do other aerobic exercises three times each week. During the 4-month program, she reduced her blood pressure from 155/90 to 130/80 and raised her sense of well-being and stamina. She maintains her exercise program and keeps her blood pressure under control by participating in water aerobics. Patricia's personal intervention in her own health profile has gone a long way to decreasing her risk for serious cardiovascular disease.

Heart health is also enhanced by the positive effect exercise has on cholesterol levels. Dr. John Duncan, associate director of the Cooper Institute for Aerobics Research in Dallas, and colleagues conducted a study to determine if the amount and speed of walking necessary to reduce the risk of cardiovascular disease in women was different from the amount and speed of walking necessary to improve cardiorespiratory fitness. Sedentary women aged 20 to 40 were divided into three walking groups and a fourth sedentary control group. Walking groups were classified as aerobic walkers (5 mph), brisk walkers (4 mph), and strollers (3 mph). All three groups walked 3 miles a day, 5 days a week for 24 weeks. At the end of the project, the women in all three groups improved their cardiorespiratory fitness. The aerobic walkers benefited most, followed by the brisk walkers and then the strollers. Interestingly, the HDL levels of all three groups of walkers improved. Considerable research documents that regular exercise moves the whole lipid profile in the right direction. A moderate amount of walking is enough to keep total cholesterol, triglycerides, and LDL cholesterol down, HDL cholesterol high, and to lower the risk of cardiovascular disease.

Exercise and Your Bones

Women are faced with increasing bone loss after menopause. A study conducted at Family Health International in Durham, North Carolina, indicates the benefit activity has on bone density. For three days, a group of 352 women aged 40 to 54 years each wore a "personal activity computer" that measured their activity levels by estimating how many calories each woman burned. The results indicated that the most active women had significantly greater bone density in their spinal vertebrae and forearms than the less active ones in the study. The greater a woman's bone density, the less likely that she will be a candidate for a fracture after menopause.

In a somewhat similar study, Dr. Everett Smith, director of the biogerontology laboratories at the University of Wisconsin's department of medicine, reported that simple exercise is adequate for maintaining healthy bone density. He found that a group of middle-aged women who regularly lifted five-pound weights for a period of four years lost bone in their arms at only half the rate expected for women who did not exercise. The results from a number of studies are very consistent and very strong. When done on a regular basis, simple weight-bearing exercises like walking and light weight lifting can help slow bone loss in postmenopausal women. This in turn reduces the risk of fracture and increases the quality of life.

More Health Benefits from Exercising

A number of additional benefits of regular exercise are sometimes over-looked. Women who exercise simply feel better. It improves their mood and lifts their self-esteem. University of Maryland researchers have found that fit seniors are better at solving arithmetic problems than those who are out of shape. Similarly, investigators at the University of Kentucky report that improving aerobic fitness increases mental skills and the ability to recall names. Exercisers also have more energy, are less likely to fatigue during their daily activities, and generally have better reaction times. They are also better able to cope with stress and anxiety both on the job and at home. Finally, regular exercisers tend to fall asleep more quickly and to sleep well. These are all qualities that should help a woman cope with transient menopause symptoms.

Recent studies also indicate that increased activity may decrease the risk of certain cancers that have a high incidence among women in their postmenopausal years. Evidence that increased exercise protects against colon cancer is especially strong. Scientists think the decrease in colon cancer is related to the fact that exercise stimulates the digestive process. This moves potential carcinogens (cancer-causing agents) through the di-gestive tract more rapidly, decreases their time in contact with the colon, and reduces the likelihood that they can promote cancer. Exercise may also reduce the risk of breast cancer and possibly other reproductive system cancers, although scientific studies are not unanimous in these findings. However, some scientists speculate that exercise alters hormone levels in a manner that wards off certain cancers.

Exercise may also help protect against noninsulin-dependent diabetes mellitus (adult onset)—another threat of the postmenopausal years. Nonin-sulin-dependent diabetes is more prevalent in sedentary than in active people. The news is also good for those who already suffer from insulin-dependent diabetes. Studies now show that exercise increases insulin sensi-tivity, so the body can use insulin more efficiently. Exercise and a sugar-restricted diet may help many noninsulin-dependent diabetic patients keep their disease under control. Exercise will probably also benefit insulin-dependent diabetic patients, but will not eliminate the need for supplemen-tal insulin. A bonus for all diabetic patients is the positive impact a regular exercise program has on peripheral circulation.

A research team from the University of California reports that an enhanced sex life may be another boon of regular exercising. The researchers persuaded a group of 78 middle-aged men to begin a regular aerobic exercise program and keep individual diaries of their sexual activity. The men's sex lives improved as their fitness levels increased. Compared to a matched sedentary control group of men, the exercisers had intercourse 30 percent more often and reportedly enjoyed it more.

Women were not included in the study, but I prefer to think that regular exercise provides similar rewards for women. If not, intercourse is still an excellent calorie-burning exercise. A 120-pound woman burns 4.2 calories per minute while making love. Playing tennis doubles only uses 4.0 calories per minute. Of course, a tennis match does last a bit longer.

Walking

Hippocrates (460–377 B.C.), the Greek physician, once wrote, "walking is man's best medicine." This bit of wisdom also applies to women and is as true today as it was over 2000 years ago. Regular walks can enhance long-term health, promote weight loss, tone muscles, and improve cardiovascular conditioning. To improve long-term health and keep muscles and joints working well into the senior years, it is simply necessary to walk a lot. According to Rob Sweetgall, president of Creative Walking Inc., in Clayton, Missouri, speed is not critical, but consistently taking regular walks is important. Walking continuously for 40 to 60 minutes is great for a woman who is in shape, but taking three 20-minute walks will use almost the same number of calories. For example, a very sedentary woman who begins walking 20 minutes every day will burn about 500 calories each week and improve her fitness level. Experts suggest that optimum gains come from walking 15 to 20 miles each week, which burns 1500 to 2000 calories.

In a recent article in *Walking*, Sweetgall outlined an excellent walking program. Although not essential to success, he recommended establishing a *target heart rate* (*THR*), which is a percentage of a person's *maximum heart rate* (*MHR*), as a goal. An appropriate THR is a little lower for long-term health (50% to 80% of MHR) and weight loss (50% to 60% of MHR) than it is for maximum benefits from cardiovascular conditioning (75% to 85% of MHR). THR is not critical for muscle toning. A THR that is 50% of your MHR should start you at a comfortable pace and get you well on your way to improving long-term health, weight loss, and cardiovascular health.

To determine your THR, take your pulse for a minute before getting out of bed in the morning. This is your *resting heart rate* (*RHR*). Then use this formula to find your THR that is 50% of your MHR:

$$[(220 - age - RHR) \times .5] + RHR = THR$$

If you are 50 years old with a RHR of 65, your THR will be:

$$[(220 - 50 - 65) \times .5] + 65 = 118$$

As fitness improves, the THR can be increased to 60 percent using the same formula.

$$[(220 - age - RHR) \times .6] + RHR = THR$$

Checking your pulse and keeping close tabs on your heart rate are not necessary since research now shows that beneficial results come with walking at almost any speed.

Walking for long-term health and walking for weight loss require similar programs. Sweetgall stresses that the important thing is to walk at a comfortable pace that you can maintain for 45 or 60 minutes. For a moderately overweight woman, walking between 3.3 mph (18-minute miles) and 3.7 mph (16-minute miles) is probably about right. A woman who needs to lose many pounds should start at a slower, more comfortable rate of 2.8 to 3.2 mph. Speed and endurance will increase with time. It is best to start at a comfortable rate and gradually work up to a goal of burning 2000 to 2500 calories per week. That amounts to two-thirds of a pound each week or 35 pounds in a year.

Muscle toning can be included in a walking program by walking up and down—hills, stairs, inclines, whatever—to tone lower body muscles. Carrying hand weights and swinging your arms tones upper body muscles. Walking for health and weight loss yields the best results if done daily. Muscle toning requires walks only 2 or 3 days each week for 20 to 40 minutes. A sedentary woman would probably benefit by first walking daily for health and/or weight loss until her stamina and endurance have improved. Then, once or twice a week, hills and weights can be added to parts of the daily walks, gradually also adding in a muscle toning program.

Cardiorespiratory conditioning can be accomplished while walking at any speed, but the brisker the walk, the greater the gain. Optimum benefits result from walking 3 or 4 times each week for 20 to 30 minutes.

Getting Started

Many women enjoy walking, but virtually any type of exercise will promote cardiovascular health before and after menopause. A study at the University of Pittsburgh included 541 healthy women aged 42 to 50. At the start of the project they had thorough physical exams and filled out questionnaires to assess their physical activity and stress levels. The women were similarly evaluated three years later. Those who had increased their physical activity had gained the least weight and had the least reduction in HDL cholesterol levels. Activities that provided these benefits varied but were equivalent to walking for 20 minutes three times a week. Other studies have confirmed the fact that intensive exercise is not necessary to provide major benefits in cardiovascular health.

The biggest obstacle to starting a regular exercise program may be mental. Once the decision to begin has been made, selecting an activity or sport should be easy. Any sport will do. A group of women in Minneapolis who were 30 to 54 years old started what they call "The World's Oldest Women's Soccer Team." The team was 6 years old and going strong when it was featured in a 1990 issue of *Women's Sports and Fitness*. Organized sports are great, but not necessary. Remember, a plan as simple as a regular walking program can provide excellent health benefits.

11

Up
in
Smoke

Smoking and Women's Health

In 1990, tobacco was singled out as the most prominent contributor to mortality in the United States. It was the underlying cause of an estimated 430,000 deaths. Yet about 46 million Americans continue to smoke. In 1985, 25 percent of all female deaths in America were related to smoking, and the numbers are rising. In 1995, smoking will contribute to 37 percent of the deaths among American women. Deaths due to lung cancer and other respiratory system diseases leap to mind and their numbers are large. However, smoking poses the threat of death from a number of other causes. The toxins from cigarette smoke have a profound effect on all the body's systems including the female reproductive system. Did you know, for example, that smoking is one of only a handful of factors that can change the timing of menopause, causing it to occur prematurely? The other primary influence that encourages an *early menopause* is diabetes mellitus which, unlike smoking, is not a matter of choice. How dramatically does smoking affect menopause? One study found that women who smoke more than 14 cigarettes each day experience menopause about 2 years earlier than women who do not smoke. The mechanism that induces early menopause and robs a woman of additional years of natural estrogen protection is not clear, but the relationship between early menopause and smoking seems undeniable. No one knows whether smoking affects the hypothalamus, pituitary, or ovaries or some combination of organs to hasten the end of the menstrual cycles and the reproductive years. Nor does anyone understand precisely how cancer of the reproductive organs is fostered by the harmful effects of smoking. However, the American Cancer Society points to smoking as the underlying cause of 30 percent of all cancers. Included among these are *ovarian cancer, cervical cancer, uterine cancer, and breast cancer*. While the exact impact of smoking on the reproductive organs is not known, overwhelming evidence indicates that smoking significantly increases a woman's risk of all types of reproductive organ cancer.

In addition to its effects on the female reproductive system, smoking also significantly increases the risk of *osteoporosis*, a major health threat to postmenopausal women. Dr. Douglas Kiel, assistant professor of internal medicine at Harvard Medical School, recently headed a team that surveyed the medical histories of almost 3000 women who took part in the Framingham Heart Study. The researchers found distinct differences in the fracture rates of smokers and nonsmokers in the group. Postmenopausal women who did not smoke and who took estrogen replacement therapy had only one-third as many fractures as smokers who had never taken estrogen. This finding is not surprising since estrogen has been shown to have a protective effect against bone loss from osteoporosis. However, it is startling that the hip fracture rate among smokers taking estrogen replacement therapy was the same as that for smokers who had never taken estrogen. The protection that estrogen normally provides against bone loss literally seems to go "up in smoke." The investigators do not know how smoking eliminates the fracture protection that estrogen replacement therapy normally provides, but they are confident that it does.

Finally, each year 500,000 women die of *cardiovascular disease*, another definite threat during the years following menopause. Over half of the deaths are due to coronary heart disease—the number-one cause of mortality among women. Smokers have a 70 percent greater death rate from coronary disease than nonsmokers. Smoking also promotes other cardiovascular diseases—*hypertension, stroke*, and *peripheral vascular disease*—and increases the risk of death from them.

The connection between smoking and cardiovascular disease is well established. Smoking lowers HDL (good cholesterol) levels, increases LDL (bad cholesterol) and triglyceride levels, increases heart rate, constricts blood vessels, increases blood pressure, and decreases the amount of oxygen that red blood cells can carry. All are factors that promote cardiovascular disease and make the health benefits of giving up smoking obvious. Researchers at Harvard University have found that men who stop smoking decrease their risk of heart attack by 50 to 70 percent. After 2 to 5 years, the risk dropped to levels comparable to those of nonsmokers. The study included only males, but similar beneficial results are expected to apply to women. Furthermore, research indicates that those who have a heart attack and continue to smoke have a 20 percent higher chance of a second heart attack than those who stop smoking. On the other hand, a number of investigations show that quitting cigarette smoking has a positive effect on the cardiovascular system. For instance, a recent report in the *Journal of the American Medical Association* assessed data from the Nurses' Health Study, a project that monitored over 50,000 women aged 45 to 67. The investigators found that women who never smoked had the lowest risk of stroke, and women who stopped smoking decreased their risk to about half that of women who continued to smoke.

The insult of tobacco on the circulatory system seems unending in promoting illnesses including *Buerger's disease*, which occurs only in smokers. It affects the small and medium arteries, veins, and nerves, commonly in the leg. The disease is characterized by inflammation and the formation of a thrombus (blood clot) that obstructs the vessels. Body parts beyond the obstruction feel cold, numb, and painful. The condition often leads to skin ulcers and progressive gangrene that usually starts in the toes or fingers. A partial recovery may occur in victims who stop smoking completely.

Evidence of the negative consequences of smoking continues to mount. Another team of investigators analyzed data from the Nurses' Health Study and found that smokers in the group were more likely to develop *cataracts* than nonsmokers. Furthermore, the risk of cataracts increased with the number of cigarettes smoked. Women in the study who smoked more than 35 cigarettes per day were considered heavy smokers and were 63 percent more likely to develop cataracts than those who never smoked. These women continued in this high-risk category even 10 years after they stopped smoking. However, light to moderate smokers who quit soon dropped to risk levels equivalent to women who had never smoked. Researchers are not sure how smoking promotes cataracts, but they know it decreases levels of certain vitamins that may play a role in keeping the lens clear. The constant and prolonged irritation of the eye by smoke may also be a factor.

Smoking can also have a devastating effect on dental and oral hygiene. Tobacco use has been directly linked to *periodontal disease*. Female smokers who are between 20 and 40 years of age are twice as likely to develop *chronic periodontitis* or *lose all of their teeth* as nonsmoking women in the same age range. Each year more than 30,000 Americans are diagnosed with *cancers of the mouth, tongue, and lips* that are directly related to tobacco use. The 5-year survival rate for patients in this category is about 50 percent.

The threat of many diseases looms large, but the danger of lung cancer is most notorious and perhaps most frightening. Since 1987, *lung cancer* has been claiming more women's lives than breast cancer, the disease that had been the leading cause of cancer deaths among women for 40 years. The rise of lung-cancer deaths among women has not been a small one. In 1950, women accounted for fewer than 20 percent of all lung-cancer deaths. Today women total over 33 percent of those dying from lung cancer. In the majority of cases, the cause is directly linked to smoking. The American Lung Association reports that people who smoke two or more packs of cigarettes each day have a 15 to 25 percent greater chance of dying from lung cancer than a nonsmoker. The devastation is not expected to end soon. Authorities estimate that over 140,000 Americans will devleop lung cancer each year during the 1990s, and, if current trends prevail, only 13 percent of the victims will still be alive 5 years after diagnosis. Perhaps the saddest statistic comes from the Environmental Protection Agency. It estimates that nearly 3 percent of cancer deaths are caused by involuntary smoking or second-hand smoke. That means about 3700 nonsmokers die each year because of exposure to someone else's smoke. An analysis of the effect of environmental smoke published in a 1994 issue of the *Journal of the American Medical Association* estimates that the risk of lung cancer increases up to 30 percent for a nonsmoking woman whose spouse is a smoker. The increased risk for lung cancer may be as high as 75 percent for a nonsmoking woman who is exposed to environmental smoke in multiple settings such as the household, workplace, and social gatherings.

Scientists have not determined exactly how smoking damages many of the reproductive organs and other body tissues to promote disease, but they do know a lot about how it modifies the respiratory system. To begin with, smoking affects the cilia-lined passageways that deliver air to the lungs. These airways are normally coated with a thin layer of mucus that traps inhaled dust and smoke particles that are swept away from the lungs by the cilia. Just one cigarette can slow the cilia. Nicotine from persistent heavy smoking paralyzes them. In the absence of functioning cilia, mucus builds up in the airways and foreign particles enter and lodge in the lungs. The loss of cilia soon begins to affect the 300 million *alveoli* or tiny elastic-like air sacs that exchange oxygen and carbon dioxide with each breath. The alveoli in smokers lungs become blackened and clogged with particles from the smoke and other environmental sources, causing them to lose resiliency and efficiency. When persistent smoking leads to lung cancer, the cancer cells grow into solid tumor masses that first interfere with lung function. Soon some of the cancer cells break off of the tumor in the lung and travel to other parts of the body; this results in dozens of secondary tumors in the brain, liver, intestines, and other body organs.

Lung cancer is not the only toll that smoking has on the respiratory system. A history of smoking also accounts for most cases of *chronic obstructive pulmonary disease* (varying combinations of emphysema, chronic bronchitis, and asthma), the fifth-leading cause of death in the United States. Quitting decreases the risk of chronic obstructive pulmonary disease and, according to a report in a 1993 issue of the *Journal of the American Medical Association*, improves pulmonary function even in those who quit after age 60. According to the U.S. Health Service, smoking is also a major contributing factor to the 1.8 million cases of sinusitis reported annually. Sinusitis occurs about 78 percent more often among smokers than among nonsmokers.

Trends in Smoking

There was a time when smoking was a habit reserved for men. Then, the story goes, around 1840, Chopin's mistress, the Baroness de Dudevant, achieved the dubious distinction of being the first women to smoke in public. Women who smoked in public were few even in 1919 when Lorilard took a bold step and used images of women smoking to market their products. The trend in women's smoking habits has certainly changed, but even in 1934 it was a noteworthy incident that Eleanor Roosevelt smoked a cigarette in public. According to best estimates, about 17 percent of the female population of the United States smoked at that time. The habit grew until 1965 when the number of smokers reached an all-time high of 34 percent of American women. We had indeed come a long way, but was there a gain? Through the 1970s and 1980s, scientific evidence accumulated implicating smoking as a significant risk factor for a number of potentially fatal diseases—many especially prevalent in the postmenopausal years. The facts were compelling enough to change the smoking habits of many women. According to the Behavioral Risk Factor Surveillance System of the Centers for Disease Control, by 1990, the number of female smokers had dropped to 21 percent, and 17 percent of all adult females were former smokers. The women who joined the ranks took a step in the right direction and reduced their risk for a number of the leading causes of death.

The changing patterns of smoking and even of acceptability of the habit are reflected in the increasing number of restaurants and public buildings that limit smoking to designated areas. For me, the most vivid perception of changing smoking patterns occurred over a period of years beginning in the late 1960s when I attended my first meeting of the American Society for Cell Biology. Through the course of the meeting, small sessions and large symposia alike seemed dominated by smokers who were encouraged by the abundance of ashtrays in virtually every area of the conference center. The beam of a 35-mm slide projector highlighted the haze of smoke that hung in the air of darkened rooms where the latest scientific data were being presented. I don't remember a distinct turning point, but during the 1970s and 1980s, scientists who made up the membership could no longer ignore the overwhelming data that smoking was directly tied to disease. At each annual meeting, the number of smokers decreased and with them the number of areas in which smoking was permitted. Smoking was essentially phased out. In the past, it was difficult for a nonsmoker to find a smoke-free area where they could catch a breath of fresh air. Now, I suspect it is difficult for the remaining smokers to find a designated smoking area where they can light up.

Unfortunately the health outlook remains grim for the many who continue to smoke. Between 1982 and 1988, the American Cancer Society undertook an enormous study of more than 1 million Americans and used the data to estimate smoking trends for all developed nations. They indicate that, if people continue smoking at current rates, one in five people now alive in developed countries will die of a cigarette-related cause—that's a total of 250 million people. In an interview published in *American Health*, Dr. Richard Peto, a professor at Oxford University in England and principal author of the study, indicated that at least one-third of all smokers die from the effects of their cigarette habit. The experts are not talking about cigarette-related deaths just among the elderly. They predict that more than half of the estimated 250 million deaths will occur among people who are 35 to 69 years of age, shortening the lives of these individuals by an average of 23 years. Because of the increase of cigarette smoking among women in recent years, it is estimated that by early next century, the habit will kill more women than men in the United States and Great Britain.

The Captivating Powers of Tobacco

It is unrealistic to believe that a person can be talked into quitting or scared into quitting by the overwhelming statistics that relate disease and death to smoking. Confronted with the facts about tobacco, cigarette smoking, and related health risks, many smokers still find it difficult or "impossible" to quit because they are addicted to nicotine. Tobacco smoke contains over 4000 chemicals, many of which are known to be harmful, but *nicotine* is the only substance that promotes chemical dependency on cigarettes. It occurs naturally in tobacco leaves and, according to the American Cancer Society, has never been found in any other plant or material. The addictive quality of nicotine stems from its action as a *psychoactive* or *mind-altering drug*. Like other psychoactive drugs (e.g., amphetamines, cocaine, and heroin), nicotine modifies brain function.

When a smoker inhales, nicotine goes first to the lungs, then enters the bloodstream. Within seven seconds, most of the nicotine has reached the brain where it mimics the action of the neurotransmitter *acetylcholine*. Like other addictive drugs, nicotine produces a feeling of euphoria that serves as a type of "reward" and encourages repeated use. Nicotine reaches a maximum concentration in the blood at about the time the cigarette butt is being crushed out. The nicotine level then begins to drop and many smokers crave more nicotine within half an hour. Even though nicotine levels drop rapidly, it takes a few cigarette-free days for nicotine to be completely cleared from the body.

While in the brain and other parts of the body, nicotine can act as a stimulant or a sedative depending on the amount taken into the body, a person's metabolism, a person's stress level, and the time of day. According to information from the American Lung Association, early in the morning nicotine acts as a stimulant to the brain and digestive tract. Later in the day, nicotine tends to act more like a sedative. Nicotine impacts a host of chemicals within the body, including neurotransmitters and hormones that regulate mood, learning, alertness, ability to concentrate, and performance.

It usually increases heart and breathing rates, constricts the diameter of peripheral blood vessels which slows down the circulation of blood, and simultaneously raises the body's demand for oxygen. This puts the body in a quandary. Blood vessels are smaller and can carry less blood. At the same time, carbon monoxide, a major component of tobacco smoke, competes with oxygen for limited space in red blood cells. The body has only one option; it compensates by pumping more blood that makes the heart work harder. In stark contrast, certain doses of nicotine have a relaxing effect, because they increase the brain's alpha waves and trigger the release of endorphins, the body's natural "feel-good" substance.

Nicotine can have many different effects. Low doses can enhance feelings of alertness or relaxation, but high ones can work as a poison. High doses of nicotine are actually used as an insecticide that works by disrupting insect neurotransmitters. A form of nicotine poisoning is experienced by most first-time smokers who become dizzy or nauseous after a few puffs. Even long-time smokers who inhale very deeply on arising in the morning or who smoke an excessive number of cigarettes in a day may experience nausea and other symptoms of nicotine poisoning. Unfortunately, the addictive quality of nicotine urges an individual to continue smoking. Those who persist in the smoking habit develop a tolerance to nicotine and require an ever-increasing number of cigarettes until they reach a nicotine level that maintains their desired level of "satisfaction." According to the American Lung Association, most smokers require a minimum of about 10 cigarettes each day to satisfy their dependence. A similar pattern of tolerance, getting used to increasing doses up to a stable level, is also characteristic of dependence on other drugs like alcohol, amphetamines, barbiturates, and narcotics.

In addition to possible nicotine addiction, most smokers develop a psychological dependence on cigarettes because they associate smoking with pleasurable activities like a cup of coffee after dinner, talking on the phone, or other forms of relaxation. The combination of physical addiction and psychological dependence make smoking a very difficult habit to break, but other factors may also influence the decision to quit smoking.

Quitting and Weight Gain

Many people, especially women, avoid attempts to break the smoking habit because they fear they will add extra pounds. Compared to the number of potentially fatal health risks promoted by smoking, the risk of gaining a few pounds on quitting would seem a minor consideration. However, many are discouraged from trying to quit by the fear of gaining weight. The tobacco industry reinforced this perception even in early advertising compaigns. For example, "Reach for a Lucky Instead of a Sweet" was the message carried by a 1928 Lucky Strike ad. Now, as then, thin well-dressed models are used in an attempt to glamorize cigarette smoking. Most investigations that address the question of weight gain after quitting find that the average person gains about 5 to 6 pounds after smoking is stopped. (It takes a gain of about 10 pounds to force a woman into the next larger dress size.) Some folks do gain more than a few pounds, but they make up a small percentage of those who quit. One study that included 20,000 men and women found that less than 4 percent of the participants who quit gained more than 20 pounds.

There are several reasons for the weight gain associated with breaking the smoking habit. For one thing, smoking can affect a person's metabolic rate. This could lead to a minor weight gain when smoking is stopped. A bigger problem is that most people tend to eat more, because food tastes better when the taste buds are no longer dulled by smoking. People sometimes nibble and snack their way through a lot of extra calories in an attempt to occupy hands and mouths with activities other than smoking. Howevever, most people do not increase other types of activities. Including an exercise program in efforts to stop smoking is a good way to burn off extra calories and to occupy the mind and body with a non-smoking-related activity.

A study reported in a recent issue of *Archives of Family Medicine* found that nicotine-containing chewing gum helped many people, especially women, kick the habit without gaining weight. Researchers at the Center for Pulmonary Disease Prevention in Palo Alto, California, compared weight changes in three groups of women who stopped smoking. One group quit smoking with the aid of chewing gum containing 2-mg doses of nicotine and a second group received gum containing 4 mg of nicotine. The third group of participants in the study received a placebo. After one cigarette-free month, the women using the placebo gained an average of three and one-half pounds, but women chewing the low-dose nicotine gum gained an average of only one pound. Women in the high-dose nicotine gum group actually lost an average of one-half pound. Three groups of men studied under the same conditions had much different results. The men in all three groups gained weight. Even the men in the group that received high-dose nicotine-containing gum gained an average of four pounds. The researchers cannot explain the differences between the sexes nor do they know if using a nicotine-containing patch will yield the same results. They also caution that ex-smokers may gain weight when they stop using the nicotine-laced gum.

There is welcome evidence that weight gains that occur after breaking the smoking habit are temporary for most people. Epidemiologist Yue Chen and his collaborators at the University of Saskatchewan followed the weight fluctuations of a group of men and women over a period of years. They found that after recently quitting smoking, men gained an average of 6.2 pounds and women gained an average of 5.5 pounds. However, *individuals who stayed off cigarettes gradually lost what they had gained*. After a period of two or more years, the former smokers had put on no more pounds than similar age-matched people who had never smoked.

Kicking the Habit

The macho Marlboro Man has disappeared from the advertising scene (in real life he died of lung cancer), but tobacco companies continue to depict smoking as a sophisticated and enjoyable pastime that is associated with thin individuals who pursue a glamorous lifestyle. In contrast, there is compelling evidence from the medical community that smoking significantly increases the risk for numerous diseases and dramatically decreases the years of one's life. While approximately 46 million Americans continue to smoke, it is promising that a 1991 Gallup poll survey found that 76 percent of them would like to quit. It is reassuring that the Centers for Disease Control reports that more than 44 million Americans had quit smoking as of 1991. Seventeen percent of all adult females were among these former smokers, and according to a 1991 Gallup poll about 76 percent of the nation's then approximately 46 million smokers indicated that they would like to quit. Even though fewer women smoke than men, the National Center for Health Statistics has reported the disturbing fact that once a woman starts to smoke, she is more likely to continue to smoke. Furthermore, there is no indication that the number of women who start to smoke is declining. The American Heart Association estimates that as many as 3000 youngsters aged 12 to 17 start smoking each day and add to the ranks of the estimated 2.2 million teenaged girls and boys who already smoke. Just as alarming is the fact that the number of women who are heavy smokers increased from 13 percent to 23 percent between 1965 and 1985. Heavy smokers are those who smoke 25 or more cigarettes a day.

Breaking the smoking habit can be difficult, but it's not impossible. The American Cancer Society estimates that about 17 million Americans try to stop smoking each year, and 1.3 million succeed in kicking the habit for good. About 65 percent of the people who set out to quit smoking start up again within the first three months, but the highest rate of relapse is actually during the first two weeks. Quitting seems to be one of those "try, try again" type of endeavors. Most people do not succeed on their first attempt, but experts do not necessarily equate relapse with failure. Instead, for many people relapse is part of a long-term quitting process that allows them to learn, try again, and eventually with repeated effort succeed. According to the American Lung Association, most people who keep trying to quit eventually do succeed in putting out their last cigarette.

As noted earlier, quitting is difficult because nicotine is an addictive drug. The absence of nicotine triggers withdrawal symptoms—a craving for nicotine, irritability, anxiety, anger, restlessness, inability to concentrate, and hunger. Ability to cope with these symptoms can make or break an attempt to quit. Consideration of how to handle withdrawal symptoms is an important issue when choosing a method for quitting.

A recent report in the *Journal of the American Medical Association* indicated that about 90 percent of successful quitters did it on their own. Most stopped smoking abruptly. However, self-help quitters do not fare as well over a 12-month period of abstinence: only 8 to 25 percent are able to refrain from lighting up again. Fewer people use an assisted method to stop smoking. This method can employ one or a combination of assisted programs, which include smoking-cessation clinics, nicotine gum, or patches, with counseling, hypnosis, or acupuncture. Those who choose an assisted program are likely to be women, who are aged 45 to 64 years, with more than a high school education, who have made several attempts to quit smoking, and who have been heavier smokers. The sustained success rate over a 12-month period is an admirable 20 to 40 percent for assisted quitters.

Smoking-cessation clinics work well for many people. Those with the greatest long-term success have a follow-up support group that continues after the initial "stop smoking" period. Nicotine-containing chewing gum or transdermal patches have both been approved for use by the Food and Drug Administration, but must be prescribed by a physician. They have been used successfully with or without attendance at a smoke-ending clinic. In either case, they are most beneficial when the prescribing physician provides the patient with adequate counseling and support.

Marion Merrell Dow manufactures *Nicorette* chewing gum in a low-dose form that contains 2 mg of nicotine and in a recently approved high dose form with 4 mg of nicotine. The user controls the dose of nicotine chewing gum on an as-needed basis (usually about 15 pieces per day). To be effective, Nicorette must be chewed slowly for about 15 chews until a peppery taste or tingling sensation is felt. Then the gum is "parked" between the cheek and the gums. When the tingling is almost gone, the user starts chewing again, until the tingling sensation returns, then she "parks" the gum once again. It takes about 30 minutes for all the nicotine to be absorbed through the mucous membranes of the mouth. Chewing too fast can create unpleasant side effects that include lightheadedness, nausea, vomiting, throat and mouth soreness, hiccups, and an upset stomach. Continuing to smoke and use the gum can intensify the side effects. However, proper use of the gum has its rewards. After two or three months, the smoker is weaned off nicotine by chewing fewer pieces of gum or chewing each piece for a shorter period of time. The gradual decrease in nicotine helps most people quit by minimizing withdrawal symptoms. The added plus mentioned above is that Nicorette helps many women control weight.

Nicotine-containing transdermal patches can also be used as a smoke-ending aide to gradually decrease nicotine dependency. Four brands of the patches are now available: *Nicoderm* from Marion Merrell Dow, *Habitrol* from Basel Pharmaceuticals, a division of CIBA-GEIGY Corporation, *Prostep* from Lederle Labs, and *Nicotrol* from Parke-Davis. Patches automatically release nicotine at a constant rate either over a 24-hour period (Nicoderm, Habitrol, and Prostep) or only during the waking hours (Nicotrol). Each brand is available in a series of two or three decreasing doses that allow patients to gradually reduce the amount of nicotine they receive over a period of weeks. The main side effect of the patch is a red, itchy skin irritation at the patch site during the first few hours after the patch is applied. This side effect is rare and is often relieved by moving the patch to a new location. Smoking while using a patch can produce symptoms of *nicotine poisoning* that can include headaches, dizziness, abdominal pain, nausea, vomiting, diarrhea, cold sweats, blurred vision, difficulty hearing, mental confusion, weakness, and fainting. If the overdose is severe, tremor, respiratory failure, low blood pressure, and prostration may occur. Success rates vary, but in general, the higher the dose of nicotine, the higher the percentage of patients who quit smoking in three to six weeks. In one study, the best results occurred when patch-users also attended weekly 45- to 60-minute group sessions to discuss their problems and reinforce their progress. The patch can curb the craving for nicotine, but the desire to quit must come from within. Dr. John Williams tells of a patient who asked him to prescribe patches to help her quit smoking. She made steady progress and in a short period of time had limited her habit to one cigarette each day. She suddenly realized that she was actually about to quit smoking. Apparently alarmed by the prospect, she removed the patch and resumed her habit! Her body was ready to give up cigarettes, but her mind was not.

If you are faced with putting down your last pack of cigarettes, be assured that it is possible to quit. I started smoking in college when advertisements applauded the glamour of smoking and many in my peer group smoked. Years later, I was smoking two packs of cigarettes a day. As a scientist, I could no longer ignore the overwhelming and compelling evidence that my smoking posed a serious health threat to my small daughter, my nonsmoking family and friends, and to myself. I was able to quit abruptly and completely over fifteen years ago. Success, however, did not come with my first attempt. It took several tries but was worth the effort. My risk for any number of diseases now falls in the range of a lifetime nonsmoker. I feel better and have more energy. Food tastes better, flowers smell better, and my house, car, clothes, and hair no longer carry the constant lingering odor of stale tobacco smoke. I truly believe quitting is possible for anyone, but I also believe that success becomes assured only after one achieves a special desire and motivation from within.

"Stop Smoking" Organizations

These national organizations have information and/or support systems that can help you stop smoking.

American Cancer Society*   800-ACS-2345
1599 Clifton Road, NE
Atlanta, GA 30329

American Heart Association*   214-373-6300
7320 Greenville Avenue
Dallas, TX 75231

American Lung Association*   212-315-8700
1740 Broadway
New York, NY 10019

Centers for Disease Control   404-639-3311
Office of Smoking and Health
1600 Clifton Road, NE, Mail Stop K-50
Atlanta, GA 30333

National Cancer Institute   800-4-CANCER
9000 Rockville Pike
Building 31, 4A-21
Bethesda, MD 20892

*Check for local chapters.

12

Looking Ahead

───────────────────────────●───────────────────────────

Trends in Women's Health Care

I t is unfortunate that research concerning women's health issues has been
sadly neglected for a long time. For obvious reasons, programs designed
to study breast and ovarian cancer have concentrated on women volunteers. However, clinical trials designed by the NIH to study many other
diseases and therapies often failed to include enough women. In 1990, the
General Accounting Office (GOA) of the federal government issued a
report that criticized this shortcoming. The GOA report opened the door
to greater awareness of the deficiencies in women's health care and was one
of many positive steps that propelled the cause of women's health issues
into the limelight. The fact remains that most trials to study causes and
treatments of heart disease, cancer, and stroke—the leading causes of death
among women—have focused on men. Physicians have used the results of
these of male-dominated studies to treat women without consideration for
gender-differences in hormone levels or other physiological factors. Yet
some of these disorders do not follow the same patterns in women as they
do in men nor do they respond to the same treatments.

Heart disease, for example, presents a striking contrast in its effects on
men and women. Women are less likely to be diagnosed as early as men.
Women are also less likely to survive a heart attack or vascular surgery
than men, and the women who do survive have poorer chances for a

satisfactory recovery. Precisely why these differences occur is a matter of debate, but preliminary explanations have been proposed. Some authorities speculate that data from the Framingham Heart Study contributed to the belief that chest pain is not a serious problem in women and encouraged physicians to ignore early warning signs. During the course of the study, investigators found that 25 percent of men who had chest pain had a heart attack within five years, while more than 80 percent of the women with chest pain never had a heart attack. Angina, the chest pain that often precedes a heart attack, was frequently disregarded by physicians and patients alike as indigestion in women. Similar pain sent most men to the emergency room.

The lack of attention to warning signs continues to be a problem, but there are also grave concerns about the necessity for better and/or different diagnostic, surgical, and therapeutic regimens for women. The medical community is now taking steps to alert women and physicians to the importance of early symptoms and to promote improved therapies. In January 1992, the National Heart, Lung, and Blood Institute convened an invitational conference, "Cardiovascular Health and Disease in Women," to focus attention on new information about health care for women patients and to evaluate gaps in current knowledge. In addition, the National Institutes of Health (NIH) are currently sponsoring the 3-year Postmenopausal Estrogen and Progestin Interventions project designed to examine the effect of hormone replacement therapy on HDL, insulin, blood pressure, and fibrinogen (a blood-clotting factor). All are considered risk indicators for cardiovascular disease. The results of this project should add greatly to the understanding of the effects of ERT on the risk of coronary heart disease.

An additional step toward greater awareness of women's health issues was made when Dr. Bernadine Healy was appointed the first female director of the NIH. The NIH also created the Office of Research on Women's Health, and, in 1991, launched the Women's Health Initiative. Between 150,000 and 160,000 women will participate in this project to study cancer, cardiovascular disease, and osteoporosis. These three concerns account for the largest number of deaths among American women. A substantial number of postmenopausal women survive cancer, cardiovascular disease, and osteoporosis only to suffer disabilities that significantly diminish their quality of life. Investigation of these serious health concerns is certainly due. In 1992, the National Cancer Institute (NCI), a division of

NIH, initiated another study designed to address these health issues. The NCI program is evaluating the efficacy of using tamoxifen to prevent breast cancer, heart attacks, and bone fractures.

Other agencies are also joining the crusade to raise the quality of health care for women. Throughout the 1990s, the Public Health Service's new Office on Women's Health is coordinating the PHS Action Plan for Women's Health. One goal is to focus attention on disorders that affect women disproportionately and to assess the underlying causes of these disorders.

Your Physician, Your Insurance, and Your Health Care

The need for improvement of women's health care has been recognized by the medical community and steps are being taken to correct omissions. Women must be willing to take advantage of the concern offered by the medical community and the attention offered by the media. However, the most important stride a women can make is to take responsibility for her own health care. This begins by wisely choosing a physician and understanding health insurance coverage. These issues can significantly influence the quality of health care received.

Selecting an appropriate physician can be more complex than one might think. For example, the number of patients a physician screens for cervical cancer by Pap smear and breast cancer by mammogram is considered an important marker when judging the quality of care received by women. A group of physicians based in Minneapolis used these criteria to determine if the sex of the physician made a difference in the delivery of health care for 97,962 women, 18 to 75 years of age, who were enrolled in a health plan in 1990. Expense was not a factor since all the women in the study had an insurance plan that covered the cost of Pap smears and mammograms. Yet the distribution of women who received these services was startling. The investigators found that women were more likely to undergo screening with Pap smears and mammograms if they saw a female physician. This was especially true if the physician was an internist or family practitioner. Young male physicians, under 38 years of age, had the lowest screening rates. However, male physicians who specialized in obstetrics and gynecology closely approached the screening rates of their female counterparts. When questioned, the most common reason women patients gave for not undergoing screening for breast and cervical cancer was that it was not offered or recommended by their physicians.

The issue of whether or not a physician offers screening tests may be further complicated for some women—especially those who do not have private insurance. Dr. J. Z. Ayanian headed a team that evaluated the relationship between the type of health insurance coverage and the clinical outcome among women with breast cancer. The concern was stimulated in part by national surveys indicating that women with private insurance are more likely to receive cancer screening than those who lack private insurance. The researchers studied 4675 women from 35 to 64 years of age who were diagnosed with invasive breast cancer between 1985 and 1987. They found that uninsured patients and those covered by Medicaid presented with more advanced breast cancer than those who were privately insured. Furthermore, uninsured and Medicaid patients were less likely to survive than privately insured women except when the cancer had already spread to distant parts of the body. The rate of insurance payment seems to contribute to the fact that privately insured patients are diagnosed earlier and enjoy a better survival rate. Medicaid reimburses health-care providers at a lower rate than other insurance organizations. Uninsured patients may pay nothing or a fraction of the amount due. The implication is that better paying patients receive better health care. The investigators concluded that women without private insurance would benefit from improved access to screening procedures and optimal therapy.

Communication Is the Key

When selecting a physician, it is important to establish that physician-patient communication is a two-way street. It is certainly a physician's responsibility to offer relevant information, screening tests, and services to a woman. On the other hand, it is a woman's responsibility to be informed, willing to request screening tests, and ready to ask questions about health concerns. The deficiencies in physician-patient communication concerning menopause and its symptoms were indicated by the results of a survey sponsored by *The North American Menopause Society* and conducted by the Gallup Organization. A total of 833 women ages 45 to 60 were polled. The results show that most women (40%) rely on the news media for information about menopause. Fewer women (36%) depend on information from their physicians while a small number of women count on friends (9%) and family members (2%) as sources. One of the biggest concerns expressed by the women was a failure on the part of the physician to address topics that women feel are major concerns. It seems many physicians spend time discussing hot flashes, night sweats, and other short-term symptoms but neglect to tell women about the dangers of osteoporosis, cardiovascular disease, or emotional symptoms. Women also expressed a concern that physicians concentrated on HRT as a means of treatment and neglected to mention any alternative therapies.

These findings put physicians in a dim light that makes them appear unresponsive to the needs of their female patients. Many in the medical community are trying to raise general awareness among health-care professionals so they present a more complete discussion of menopause with their patients. Some physicians may deserve to be admonished for not providing enough information to patients in their perimenopause years. However, it is probably not efficient or necessary for every physician to tell every woman about all the possible menopause symptoms. A woman who is overcome by hot flashes and concerned about a family history of heart disease probably does not need a lengthy lecture on other possible menopause symptoms like itchy eyes, crawly skin, and migraines.

Most physicians are happy to address a patient's concerns but must first be aware of those concerns. It is a good idea to take a written list of physical complaints and questions when seeing the doctor. It is not fair to make a doctor's appointment to address one problem and then expect the physician to guess at other questions you may like to have answered. The responsibility for physician-patient communication needs to be equally shared.

We should be encouraged by the medical community's increasing awareness of women's health-care issues, particularly problems promoted by decreasing estrogen levels at menopause. Women no longer need to "suffer through" the transient symptoms of menopause or feel helpless in the face of increased risks for long-term consequences like osteoporosis and cardiovascular disease. A turning point has been reached. The stage is now set for women to become increasingly active participants in their own health-care management and to look forward to many healthy years of postmenopausal life.

SELECTED SOURCES

•

Chapter 1
The Chemistry
of Love

Cutler, Winnifred B. 1991. *Love Cycles: The Science of Intimacy*. New York: Villard
Books.

Fisher, Helen E. 1992. *Anatomy Of Love. The Natural History Of Monogamy,
Adultery, and Divorce*. New York: W. W. Norton & Co.

Kelley, Dennis D. 1985. Sexual Differentiation of the Nervous System. In Eric R.
Kandel and J. H. Schwartz (Eds.), *Principles of Neural Science*, 2nd ed. New
York: Elsevier.

McEwen, Bruce S. 1976. Interactions between hormones and nerve tissue. *Scientific
American* 235(1):48–58.

Money, John. 1986. *Venuses Penuses, Sexology, Sexosophy and Exigency Theory*.
Buffalo, N.Y.: Prometheus Books.

Sherwin, Barbara B. 1991. The impact of different doses of estrogen and progestin
on mood and sexual behavior in postmenopausal women. *Journal of Clinical
Endocrinology and Metabolism* 72(2):336–343.

Snyder, Soloman H. 1985. The molecular basis of communication between cells.
Scientific American (October):132–141

Toran-Allerand, C. D. 1978. Gonadal hormones and brain development: Cellular
aspects of sexual differentiation. *American Zoologist* 18:553–565.

Toran-Allerand, C. D. 1984. On the genesis of sexual differentiation of the central
nervous system: Morphognetic consequences of steroidal exposure and pos-

sible role of α-fetoprotein. In G. J. De Vries, J. P. C. DeBruin, H. B. M. Uylings, and M. A. Corner (Eds.), *Sex Differences in the Brain: The Relation Between Structure and Function. Progress in Brain Research* 61:63–98.

Walsh, Anthony. 1991. *The Science Of Love: Understanding Love and its Effects on Mind and Body.* Buffalo, N.Y.: Prometheus Books.

Chapter 2
Hormone Cycles

Baird, David T. and Anna F. Glasier. 1993. Hormonal contraception. *New England Journal of Medicine* 328(21):1543–1548.

Budoff, P. W. 1983. *No More Menstrual Cramps and Other Good News.* New York: G. P. Putnam's Sons.

Camp, J. 1974. *Magic, Myth and Medicine.* New York: Taplinger Publishing Co., Inc.

Dyer, K. A. 1990. Curiosities of contraception: a historical perspective. *Journal of the American Medical Association* 264:2818–2819.

Gannon, Linda R. 1985. *Menstrual Disorders and Menopause.* New York: Praeger Press.

Glasier, Anna, K. J. Thong, M. Dewar, M. Mackie, and D. T. Baird. 1992. Mifepristone (RU486) compared with high-dose estrogen and progestogen for emergency postcoital contraception. *New England Journal of Medicine* 327(15):1041–1044.

Healy, David L., A. O. Trounson, and A. N. Andersen. 1994. Female infertility: causes and treatment. *The Lancet* 343:1539–1544.

Mosher, W. D. and W. F. Pratt. 1990. Fecundity and infertility in the United States, 1965–1988: advanced data from vital and health statistics. Hyattsville: National Center for Health Statistics.

Peyron, Remi, E. Aubény, V. Targoz, L. Silvestre, M. Renault, F. Elkik, P. Leclerc, A. Ulmann, and E. Baulieu. 1993. Early termination of pregnancy with mifepristone (RU486) and the orally active prostaglindin misoprostol. *New England Journal of Medicine* 328(21):1509–1513.

Preti, G., W. B. Cutler, C. M. Christensen, H. Lawley, G. R. Huggins, and C. R. Garcia. 1987. Human axillary extracts: analysis of compounds from samples which influence menstrual timing. *Journal of Chemical Ecology* 13:717–731.

Wasserman, P. M. 1987. The Biology and Chemistry of Fertilization. *Science* 235: 553–559.

Chapter 3
Making Sense of the
Menopause Myths

Brecher, Edward M. 1984. *Love, Sex, and Aging.* Boston: Little, Brown.

Breslau, N., M. M. Kilbey, and P. Andreski. 1993. Nicotine dependence and major depression: New evidence from a prospective investigation. *Archives of General Psychiatry* 50:31–35.

Cotton, P. 1994. Constellation of risks and processes seen in search for Alzheimer's clues. *Journal of the American Medical Association* 271:89–91.

Demers, Laurence M. (Ed.). 1989. *Premenstrual, Postpartum, and Menopausal Mood Disorders*. Baltimore: Urban and Schwarzenberg.

Formanek, Ruth (Ed.). 1990. *The Meanings of Menopause: Historical, Medical, and Clinical Perspectives*. Hillsdale, N.J.: Analytic Press.

Greene, John G. 1984. *The Social and Psychological Origins of the Climacteric Syndrome*. Brookfield, VT.: Gower Press.

Horton, J. A. (Ed.). 1992. *The Women's Health Data Book*. New York: Elsevier.

Jackson, S. W. 1986. *Melancholia And Depression*. New Haven, Conn.: Yale University Press.

Kagan, Julia and Jo David. 1991. The facts of life: What every woman over 35 needs to know about her body. *McCall's Magazine* June:60 (8 pp.).

Køster, A. and K. Garde. 1993. Sexual desire and menopausal development. A prospective study of Danish women born in 1936. *Maturitas* 16:49–60.

London, S. N. and C. B. Hammond. 1986. The Climacteric. In: D. N. Danforth and J. R. Scott (Eds.). *Obstetrics and Gynecology*. Philadelphia: J. B. Lippincott Co.

McCraw, R. K. 1991. Psychosexual changes associated with the perimenopausal period. *Journal of Nurse Midwifery* 36:17–24.

McKinlay, S. M., D. J. Brambilla, and J. G. Posner. 1992. The normal menopause transition. *Maturitas* 14:103–115.

Myers, L. S., J. Dixen, D. Morrissette, M. Carmichael, and J. M. Davidson. 1990. Effects of estrogen, androgen, and progestin on sexual psychophysiology and behavior in postmenopausal women. *Journal of Clinical Endocrinology and Metabolism* 70(4):1124–1131.

Parazzini, F., E. Negri, and C. La Vecchia. 1992. Reproductive and general lifestyle determinants of age at menopause. *Maturitas* 15:141–149.

Raymond, C. A. 1988. Studies question the role of menopause in women's emotional distress. *Journal of the American Medical Association* 259(24):3522–3523.

Sarrel, P. M. 1990. Sexuality and menopause. *Obstetrics & Gynecology* 75(4):26S–30S.

Toran-Allerand, C. D., R. C. Miranda, W. D. L. Bentham, F. Sohrabji, T. J. Brown, R. B. Hochberg, and N. J. MacLusky. 1992. Estrogen receptors colocalize with low-affinity nerve growth factor receptors in cholinergic neurons of the basal forebrain. *Proceedings of the National Academy of Science* 89:4668–4672.

Wiklund, I., J. Holst, J. Karlberg, L.-A. Mattsson, G. Samsioe, K. Sandin, M.

Uvebrant, and B. von Schoultz. 1992. A new methodological approach to the evaluation of quality of life in postmenopausal women. *Maturitas* 14: 211–224.

Chapter 4
More Changes

Budoff, Penny W., 1983. No More Hot Flashes and Other Good News. New York: G.P. Putnam's Sons.

Cady, R. K., J. K. Wendt, J. R. Kirchner, J. D. Sargent, J. F. Rothrock, and H. Skaggs, Jr. 1991. Treatment of acute migraine with subcutaneous sumatriptan. *Journal of the American Medical Association* 265:2831–2835.

Chalker, Rebecca and Kristene E. Whitmore. 1990. *Overcoming Bladder Disorders*. Harper and Row. New York.

Cutler, Winnifred B. 1991. *Love Cycles: The Science of Intimacy*. New York: Villard Books.

Fantl, J. A., J. F. Wyman, D. K. McClish, S. W. Harkins, R. K. Elswick, J. R. Taylor, E. C. Hadley. 1991. Efficacy of bladder training in older women with urinary incontinence. *Journal of the American Medical Association* 265(5):609–613.

Felson, D. T., D. Sloutskis, J. J. Anderson, J. M. Anthony and D. P. Kiel. 1991. Thiazide diuretics and the risk of hip fracture. Results from The Framingham Study. *Journal of the American Medical Association* 265(3): 370–373.

Flint, Marcha, Fredi Kronenberg, and Wolf Utian (Eds.). 1990. *Multidisciplinary Perspectives on Menopause*. New York: New York Academy of Sciences.

Freedman, R. R., S. Woodward, and S. C. Sabharwal. 1990. α_2-adrenergic mechanism in menopausal hot flushes. *Obstetrics and Gynecology* 76:573–578.

Gannon, Linda R. 1985. *Menstrual Disorders and Menopause*. New York: Praeger Press.

Gosden, R. G., 1985. *Biology of Menopause: The Causes and Consequences of Ovarian Ageing*. Orlando: Academic Press.

Keyser, H. H. 1984. *Women Under the Knife*. New York: Warner Books.

Lenton, E. A., L. Sexton, S. Lee, and I. D. Cooke. 1988. Progressive changes in LH and FSH and LH: FSH ratio in women throughout reproductive life. *Maturitas* 10:35–43.

Metka, M., H. Enzelsberger, W. Knogler, B. Schurz, and H. Aichmair. 1991. Ophthalmic complaints as a climacteric symptom. *Maturitas* 14:3–8.

Mishell, Daniel R. (Ed.). 1987. *Menopause: Physiology and Pharmacology*. Chicago: Year Book Medical Publishers.

Pearlman, J. 1990. Migraine Salvation. *Health* (April):52–57 & 83–84.

Notelovitz, M. and D. Tonnessen. 1993. *Estrogen: Yes or No?* New York: St. Martin's Paperbacks.

Ravnikar, V. 1990. Physiology and treatment of hot flushes. *Obstetrics and Gynecology* 75(4):3s–7s.

Raz, R. and W. E. Stamm. 1993. A controlled trial of intravaginal estriol in postmenopausal women with recurrent urinary tract infections. *New England Journal of Medicine* 329(11):753–756.

Rekers, H., A. C. Drogendijk, H. A. Valkenburg, and F. Riphagen. 1992. The menopause, urinary incontinence and other symptoms of the genitourinary tract. *Maturitas* 15:101–111.

Rozenberg, S., D. Bosson, A. Peretz, A. Caufriez, and C. Robyn. 1988. Serum levels of gonadotrophins and steroid hormones in the post-menopause and later life. *Maturitas* 10:215–224.

Stewart, W. F., R. B. Lipton, D. D. Celentano, and J. L. Reed. 1992. Prevalence of migraine headache in the United States. *Journal of the American Medical Association* 267:64–69.

U. S. Department of Health and Human Services. 1991. Unrinary incontinence among hospitalized persons aged 65 years and older—United States, 1984–1987. *Morbidity and Mortality Weekly Report* 40(26):433–436.

U. S. Department of Health and Human Services. 1993. Migraine drug approved. *FDA Consumer* 27:2–3.

Utian, W. H. and Ruth S. Jacobowitz. 1990. *Managing Your Menopause*. New York: Prentice-Hall Press.

Welch, K. M. A. 1993. Drug therapy of migraine. *New England Journal of Medicine* 329:1476–1484.

Chapter 5
Menopause Before
Your Time

Broder, S. 1992. Rapid Communication—The Bethesda System for reporting cervical/vaginal cytological diagnoses. *Journal of the American Medical Association* 267(14):1892.

Carlson, K. J., D. H. Nichols, and I. Schiff. 1993. Indications for Hysterectomy. *New England Journal of Medicine* 329:856–860.

Cutler, Winnifred B. 1988. *Hysterectomy: Before and After*. New York: Harper & Row, Publishers.

Farley, D. 1993. Endometriosis—Painful, but treatable. *FDA Consumer* January–February, 1993:25–27.

Healey, D. L., H. G. Burger, P. Mamers, T. Jobling, M. Bangah, M. Quinn, P. Grant, A. J. Day, R. Rome, and J. J. Campbell. 1993. Elevated serum inhibin concentrations in postmenopausal women with ovarian tumors. 329:1539–1542.

Hummel, S. J. and M. Lindquist. 1992. *If It Runs in Your Family: Ovarian and Uterine Cancer*. New York: Bantam Books.

Kjerulff, Kristen, P. Langenberg and G. Guzinski. 1993. The socioeconomic correlates of hysterectomies in the United States. *American Journal of Public Health* 83:106–108.

Narod, Steven A., Jean Feunteun, Henry T. Lynch, Patrice Watson, Theresa Conway, Jane Lynch, and Gilbert M. Lenoir. 1991. Familial breast-ovarian cancer locus on chromosome 17q12–q23. *Lancet* 338:82–83.

Rudy, D. R. and I. M. Bush. 1992. Hysterectomy and sexual dysfunction: You can help. *Patient Care* September 30, 1992:67–70.

Segal, M. 1992. Ovarian cancer–Early detection elusive. *FDA Consumer* November, 1992:15–18.

Segal, M. 1992. Ovarian cancer–Today's treatment, tomorrow's hope. *FDA Consumer* December, 1992:13–15.

Tobin, M. J. 1992. Why aren't more FPs seeing endometriosis? *Endometriosis Today* 1(1):1–2.

U. S. Centers for Disease Control. 1993. More professional women die from breast cancer. *Cancer Researcher* 27:4.

Voight, Lynda F., Noel S. Weiss, Joseph Chu, Janet R. Daling, Barbara McKnight, and Gerald van Belle. 1991. Progestagen supplementation of exogenous oestrogens and risk of endometrial cancer. *Lancet* 338:274–277.

Williamson, M. L. 1992. Sexual adjustment after hysterectomy. *Journal of Gynecologic and Neonatal Nursing* 21(1):42–47.

Chapter 6
The Silent
Epidemic

Cauley, J. A., J. P. Gutai, L. H. Kuller, D. LeDonne, R. B. Sandler, D. Sashin, and J. G. Powell. 1988. Endogenous estrogen levels and calcium intakes in postmenopausal women. Relationships with cortical bone measures. *Journal of the American Medical Association* 260:3150–3155.

Christiansen, Claus, Merete S. Christensen, and I. Transbøl. 1981. Bone mass in postmenopausal women after withdrawal of oestrogen/gestagen replacement therapy. *Lancet* 28:459–461.

Cooper, Kenneth H. 1989. *Preventing Osteoporosis*. New York: Bantam Books.

Drinkwater, B. L., B. Bruemner, C. H. Chesnut III. 1990. Menstrual history as a determinant of current bone density in young athletes. *Journal of the American Medical Association* 263:545–548.

Greenspan, S. L., E. R. Myers, L. A. Maitland, N. M. Resnick, and W. C. Hayes. 1994. Fall severity and bone mineral density as risk factors for hip fracture in ambulatory elderly. *Journal of the American Medical Association* 271:128–133.

Hay, E. K. 1991. That old hip. The osteoporosis process. *Nurs. Clin. of North America* 26:43–51.

Lindsay, R. and J. F. Tohme. 1990. Estrogen treatment of patients with established postmenopausal osteoporosis. *Obstetrics & Gynecology* 76:290–295.

Marslew, U., K. Overgaard, B. J. Riis, and C. Christiansen. 1992. Two new combinations of estrogen and progestogen for prevention of postmenopausal bone loss: long-term effects on bone, calcium and lipid metabolism, climacteric symptoms, and bleeding. *Obstetrics & Gynecology* 79:202–210.

McIlwain, Harris H., Debra F. Bruce, Joel C. Silverfield, and Michael C. Burnette, 1988. *Osteoporosis: Prevention, Management, Treatment*. New York: John Wiley and Sons, Inc.

Shangold, M., R. W. Rebar, A. C. Wentz, and I. Schiff. 1990. Evaluation and management of menstrual dysfunction in athletes. *Journal of the American Medical Association* 263:1665–1669.

Chapter 7
The Heart of
the Matter

Barrett-Connor, E. and T. L. Bush. 1991. Estrogen and coronary heart disease in women. *Journal of the American Medical Association* 265:1861–1867.

Brown, M. S. and J. L. Goldstein. 1984. How LDL receptors influence cholesterol and atherosclerosis. *Scientific American* 251(November):58–66.

Browner, W. S., J. Westenhouse, and J. A. Tice. 1991. What if Americans ate less fat? A quantitative estimate of the effect on mortality. *Journal of the American Medical Association* 265:3285–3291.

Cimons, M. 1993. Special report. Don't die! *Rodale's Healthy Women* Summer 1993: 56–67.

Gotto, A. M., J. C. LaRosa, D. Hunninghake, S. M. Grundy, P. W. Wilson, T. B. Clarkson, J. W. Hay, D. S. Goodman. 1990. Special Report. The Cholesterol Facts. A summary of the evidence relating dietary fat, serum cholesterol, and coronary heart disease. A Joint Statement by the American Heart Association and the National Heart, Lung, and Blood Institute. *Circulation* 81(5):1721–1733.

Healy, Bernadine. 1991. Preventing heart disease in women. *Journal of the American Medical Association* 266(4):565–566.

Horton, J. A. 1992. *The Women's Health Data Book*. New York: Elsevier.

Kowalski, R. E. 1992. *8 Steps to a Healthy Heart*. New York: Warner Books.

Manson, J. E., M. J. Stampfer, G. A. Colditz, W. C. Willett, B. Rosner, F. E. Speizer, C. H. Hennekens. 1991. A prospective study of aspirin use and primary prevention of cardiovascular disease in women. *Journal of the American Medical Association* 266(4):521–527.

Martin, K. A. and M. W. Freeman. 1993. Postmenopausal hormone-replacement therapy. *New England Journal of Medicine* 328(15):1115–1117.

Nabulshi, A. A., A. R. Folsom, A. White, W. Patsch, G. Heiss, K. K. Wu, and M. Szklo. 1993. Association of hormone-replacement therapy with various cardiovascular risk factors in postmenopausal women. *New England Journal of Medicine* 328(15):1069–1075.

Stampfer, M. J. and G. A. Colditz. 1991. Estrogen replacement therapy and coronary heart disease: a quantitative assessment of the epidemiologic evidence. *Preventive Medicine* 20(1):47–63.

Vandenbroucke, J. P. 1991. Postmenopausal oestrogen and cardioprotection. *Lancet* 337:833–834.

Wenger, N. K., L. Speroff, and B. Packard. 1993. Cardiovascular health and disease in women. *New England Journal of Medicine* 329(4):247–256.

Chapter 8
Hormone
Replacement
Therapy

Abrams, J. 1991. Estrogen replacement for the 1990s. *New England Journal of Medicine* 88(3):177–179.

Arafat, E. S., J. T. Hargrove, W. S. Maxson, D. M. Desiderio, A. C. Wentz, and R. N. Andersen. 1988. Sedative and hypnotic effects of oral administration of micronized progesterone may be mediated through its metabolites. *American Journal of Obstetrics and Gynecology* 159:1203–1209.

Belchetz, P. E. 1994. Hormonal treatment of postmenopausal women. *New England Journal of Medicine* 330:1062–1071.

Davidson, M., K. R. Epstein, M. A. Freedman, G. I. Gorodeski, and N. K. Wenger. 1993. Established cardiovascular disease—does HRT offer benefits? *Menopause Management* 11(9):10–16.

Kadri, A. Z. 1991. Hormone replacement therapy—a survey of perimenopausal women in a community setting. *British Journal of General Practice* 41:109–112.

Katzenellenbogen, Benita S. 1991. Antiestrogen resistance: mechanisms by which breast cancer cells undermine the effectiveness of endocrine therapy. *Journal of the National Cancer Institute* 83:1434–1435.

Martin, K. A. and M. W. Freeman. 1993. Postmenopausal hormone-replacement therapy. *New England Journal of Medicine* 328(15):1115–1117.

Nachtigall, L. E. 1990. Enhancing patient compliance with hormone replacement therapy at menopause. *Obstetrics & Gynecology* 75(S):77S–80S.

Nachtigall, Lila E. and Joan R. Heilman. 1991. *Estrogen*. New York: Harper Perennial.

Sitruk-Ware, R. 1992. Estrogen, progestins and breast cancer risk in postmenopausal women: state of the ongoing controversy in 1992. *Maturitas* 15:129–139.

Stumpf, P. G. 1990. Pharmocokinetics of estrogen. *Obstetrics & Gynecology* 75(4): 9S–14S.

Voigt, L. F., N. S. Weiss, J. Chu, J. R. Daling, B. McKnight, and G. van Belle. 1991. Progestagen supplementation of exogenous oestrogens and risk of endometrial cancer. *Lancet* 338:274–277.

Wiklund, I., G. Berg, M. Hammar, J. Karlberg, R. Lindgren, and K. Sandin. 1992. Long-term effect of transdermal hormonal therapy on aspects of quality of life in postmenopausal women. *Maturitas* 14:225–236.

Zumoff, B. 1993. Hormone replacement and cardiovascular risk factors (Correspondence). *New England Journal of Medicine* 329(14):1041.

Chapter 9
You Are What
You Eat

Barrett-Connor, E., J. C. Chang, and S. L. Edelstein. 1994. Coffee-associated osteoporosis offset by daily milk consumption. *Journal of the American Medical Association* 271:280–283.

Browner, W. S., J. Westenhouse, and J. A. Tice. 1991. What if Americans ate less fat? A quantitative estimate of the effect on mortality. *Journal of the American Medical Association* 265(24):3285–3291.

Davidson, M. H., L. D. Dugan, J. H. Burns, J. Bova, K. Story, and K. B. Drennan. 1991. The hypocholesterolemic effects of β-glucan in oatmeal and oat bran. *Journal of the American Medical Association* 265(14):1833–1839.

Grundy, S. M. 1990. Cholesterol and coronary heart disease. Future directions. *Journal of the American Medical Association* 264(23):3053–3059.

Horton, J. A. (Ed) 1992. Addictive Behaviors. In: *The Women's Health Book. A Profile of Women's Health in the United States*. New York: Elsevier.

Hunter, D. J., J. E. Manson, G. A. Colditz, M. J. Stampfer, B. Rosner, C. H. Hennekens, F. E. Speizer, and W. C. Willett. 1993. A prospective study of the intake of vitamins C, E, and A and the risk of breast cancer. *New England Journal of Medicine* 329(4):234–240.

Johnson, K. and E. W. Kligman. 1992. Preventive nutrition: An 'optimal' diet for older adults. *Geriatrics* 47(10):56–60.

Johnson, K. and E. W. Kligman. 1992. Preventive nutrition: Disease-specific dietary interventions for older adults. *Geriatrics* 47(11):39–49.

Losing weight. What works. What doesn't. 1993. *Consumer Reports*. June 1993: 347–357.

McGinnis, J. M. and W. H. Foege. 1993. Actual causes of death in the United States. *Journal of the American Medical Association* 270(18):2207–2212.

Rimm, E. B., M. J. Stampfer, A. Ascherio, E. Giovannucci, G. A. Colditz, and W. C. Willett. 1993. Vitamin E consumption and the risk of coronary heart disease in men. *New England Journal of Medicine* 328(20):1450–1456.

Stampfer, M. J., C. H. Hennekens, J. E. Manson, G. A. Colditz, B. Rosner, and W. C. Willett. 1993. Vitamin E consumption and the risk of coronary disease in women. *New England Journal of Medicine* 328(20):1444–1449.

Steinberg, D. 1993. Antioxidant vitamins and coronary heart disease. *New England Journal of Medicine* 328(20):1487–1489.

Chapter 10
Survival of
the Fittest

Cahill, K. M. 1992. Pressure treatment. How exercise can help you control your blood pressure. *Walking* May/June:17–18.

Curfman, G. D. 1993. The health benefits of exercise. A critical reappraisal. *New England Journal of Medicine* 328(8):574–576.

Duncan, J. J., N. F. Gordon, and C. B. Scott. 1991. Women walking for health and fitness. How much is enough? *Journal of the American Medical Association* 266(23):3295–3299.

Fiatrone, M. A., E. F. O'Neill, N. D. Ryan, K. M. Clements, G. R. Solares, M. E. Nelson, S. B. Roberts, J. J. Kehayias, L. A. Lipsitz, and W. J. Evans. 1994. Exercise training and nutritional supplementation for physical frailty in very elderly people. *New England Journal of Medicine* 330:1769–1775.

Karvenen, K., M. McCloy, and M. Kort. 1991. Myth busters. *Women's Sports and Fitness* October:48–56.

Paffenbarger, R. S., R. T. Hyde, A. L. Wing, I-M. Lee, D. L. Jung, and J. B. Kampert. 1993. The association of changes in physical-activity level and other lifestyle characteristics with mortality among men. *New England Journal of Medicine* 328(8):538–545.

Sandvik, L., J. Erikssen, E. Thaulow, G. Erikssen, R. Mundal, and K. Rodahl. 1993. Physical fitness as a predictor of mortality among healthy, middle-aged Norwegian men. *New England Journal of Medicine* 328(8):533–537.

Shephard, R. J. 1993. Exercise and aging: Extending independence in older adults. *Geriatrics* 48(5):61–64.

Sweetgall, R. 1993. A custom fit. How to design the perfect personal walking program. *Walking* (March/April) 8:37–44.

Chapter 11
Up in Smoke

American Cancer Society: 1991. *Cancer Facts & Figures–1991.* New York: American Cancer Society.

American Lung Association: 1985. *Second-Hand Smoke: Take a Look at the Facts.* New York: American Lung Association.

Centers for Disease Control and Prevention. 1993. Cigarette smoking among adults—United States. *Morbidity and Mortality Weekly Report* 42:230–233.

Chesebro, M. J. 1988. Passive smoking. *American Family Physician* 37(5):212–218.

Ernster, V. L. 1985. Mixed messages for women: A social history of cigarette smoking and advertising. *New York State Journal of Medicine* 85:335–340.

Fiore, M. C., S. S. Smith, D. E. Jorenby, and T. B. Baker. 1994. The effectiveness of the nicotine patch for smoking cessation—a meta-analysis. *Journal of the American Medical Association* 271:1940–1947.

Fontham, E. T. H., P. Correa, P. Reynolds, A. Wu-Williams, P. A. Buffler, R. S. Greenberg, V. W. Chen, T. Alterman, P. Boyd, D. F. Austin, and J. Liff. 1994. Environmental tobacco smoke and lung cancer in nonsmoking women. *Journal of the American Medical Association* 271:1752–1759.

Higgins, M. W., P. L. Enright, R. A. Kronmal, M. B. Schenker, H. Anton-Culver, and M. Lyles. 1993. Smoking and lung function in elderly men and women. *Journal of the American Medical Association* 269(21):2741–2748.

Hurt, R. D., L. C. Dale, P. A. Fredrickson, C. C. Caldwell, G. A. Lee, K. P. Offord, G. G. Lauger, Z. Marušić, L. W. Neese, and T. G. Lundberg. 1994. Nicotine patch therapy for smoking cessation combined with physician advice and nurse follow-up—one-year outcome and percentage of nicotine replacement. *Journal of the American Medical Association* 271:595–600.

Kaufman, N. J. 1994. Smoking and young women—the physician's role in stopping an equal opportunity killer. *Journal of the American Medical Association* 271:629–630.

Kawachi, I., G. A. Colditz, M. J. Stampfer, W. C. Willett, J. E. Manson, B. Rosner, F. E. Speizer, and C. H. Hennekens. 1993. Smoking cessation and decreased risk of stroke in women. *Journal of the American Medical Association* 269(2):232–236.

Kenford, S. L., M. C. Fiore, D. E. Jorenby, S. S. Smith, D. Wetter, and T. B. Baker. 1994. Predicting smoking cessation—who will quit with and without the nicotine patch. *Journal of the American Medical Association* 271:589–594.

Lewis, R. 1992. Prescriptions to help smokers quit. *FDA Consumer* December:16–21.

Sennott-Miller, L. and E. W. Kligman. 1992. Healthier lifestyles: How to motivate older patients to change. *Geriatrics* 47(12):52–59.

Office on Smoking and Health. National Center for Chronic Disease Prevention and Health Promotion, CDC. Strategies-United States. *Journal of the American Medical Association* 268(13):1645–1646.

Orleans, C. T., N. Resch, E. Noll, M. K. Keintz, B. K. Rimer, T. V. Brown, and T. M. Snedden. 1994. Use of transdermal nicotine in a state-level prescription plan for the elderly—a first look at 'real world' patch users. *Journal of the American Medical Association* 271:601–607.

Satcher, D. and M. Eriksen. 1994. The paradox of tobacco control (editorial). *Journal of the American Medical Association* 271:627–628.

Timmreck, T. C. and J. F. Randolph. 1993. Smoking cessation: Clinical steps to improve compliance. *Geriatrics* 48(4):63–70.

U. S. Department of Health and Human Services. 1989. *The Health Consequence of Smoking: Nicotine Addiction. A Report of the Surgeon General.* U.S. Department of Health and Human Services, Public Health Service. Office on Smoking and Health.

U. S. Department of Health and Human Services: *Smoking, Tobacco, and Health: A Fact Book.* U.S. Department of Health and Human Services, Public Health Service, Office on Smoking and Health. DHHS Publication No. (CDC) 87–8397 (Revised 10/89).

U. S. Department of Health and Human Services. 1990. Trends in lung cancer incidence and mortality—United States, 1980–1987. *Morbidity and Mortality Weekly Report* 39:875–878.

Chapter 12
Looking
Ahead

Aburdene, P. and J. Naisbitt. 1992. *Megatrends for Women.* New York: Villard Books.

Ayanian, J. Z., B. A. Kohler, T. Abe, and A. M. Epstein. 1993. The relation between health insurance coverage and clinical outcomes among women with breast cancer. *New England Journal of Medicine* 329:326–331.

Clinician-patient dialogue about menopause: Is there room for improvement? 1993. *Menopause Management* 2(9):22–23.

Doress, Paula B. and Diana L. Siegel. 1987. *Ourselves Growing Older: Women Aging with Knowledge and Power*. New York: Simon and Schuster.

Foley, D. and E. Nechas. 1993. It's not all in your head. *Rodale's Healthy Woman* Winter:34–39.

Lurie, N., J. Slater, P. McGovern, J. Ekstrum, L. Quam, and K. Margolis. 1993. Preventive care for women Does the sex of the physician matter? *New England Journal of Medicine* 329(7):478–482.

INDEX